# CRY BABEL

CRYSTAL BELL

# CRY BABEL

*The Nightmare of Aphasia
and a Courageous Woman's
Struggle to Rebuild Her Life*

*April Oursler Armstrong*

*Doubleday & Company, Inc., Garden City, New York* 1979

ISBN: 0-385-13529-7
Library of Congress Catalog Card Number: 77-26511
Copyright © 1979 by April Oursler Armstrong
Printed in the United States of America
First Edition

For my son Kevin,
who was baptized and named for the poet Caedmon,
called to sing by an angel,
this book is dedicated
through the living Heart.

# INTRODUCTION

"My God, why? And what do You want me to do?"

In that tone is everything: fear, awe, sadness, pain, excitement, disenchantment, despair, help, release, gladness, joy, faith, love. And above all, hope.

The deepest level of you is a joyful anguish of being alive. As for being alive, that includes every feeling, every awareness. I never really understood that until I also realized I was handicapped, and was being a child at last.

In 1972 an aneurysm on an artery of my brain ruptured. With surgery the artery was physically restored. I suffered aphasia, a medical term for "loss of language." All my language skills—speech, writing, understanding, and reading—were gone. I was close to global aphasia, but I could remember people, and there were seven real words left in my brain. Of that small group the two most important were "April" and "God."

I needed intense physical therapy. The left side of the brain was the site of the hemorrhage, and the right side of the body was numb, so I was unable to walk correctly, and my visual field was confused. I did not see the world the same way as before.

There are a million Americans with aphasia. Some have it from strokes, some from accidents in cars, some from bullets, and some from aneurysms. They are handicapped, and they are prisoners in many ways.

I'm lucky. I can now communicate, because I have learned how to talk again. But, for the early months after the operation, many people believed I no longer was myself. They knew me to be handicapped by the aneurysm, the operation, and aphasia. They silently believed I had lost all my marbles. Only I knew I was still myself. Those with aphasia are prisoners, jailed by the so-called normal people, who are too scared to communicate with the disabled ones.

With charity, there is a key to unlock the vision of human life. My first time around, I, like everybody else, thought I had the key. I had been kind, trustful, helpful to all—or so I thought. But with aphasia it's easier to see the world. Like it or not, we are childlike. Emotionally, mentally, and spiritually, we are naked.

In the Bible, in Genesis, is the story of human life in which all men had but one language. Men thought they were so great and were so busy making a skyscraper that they forgot to remember God. So the Lord came down to earth and changed men so they could not understand each other and communicate. People were separated by languages.

In the beginning of aphasia, my words were a babble of nonsense. But, inside myself, I understood. Everyone has to learn the language of charity. All people, including the so-called normal people, are born handicapped. Everyone is normal. Everyone is handicapped. We are all in one boat with God.

I've been on both sides in the boat. And I hope to be able to translate the language barrier of Babel.

Years have passed. I still have problems with language skills. I went to school to speech pathologists. I have some trouble spelling, and with arithmetic. With crossword puzzles I'm up to fourth grade—I who used to love the Sunday New York *Times*. My idioms are doing better. I read fairly well, but reading out loud is sometimes unreal. Proper names are hard. Show me the name written down and I understand. After all, I am still learning to know what a whisk broom is called. (I do know how to use it.) I seldom can understand a joke said, or explained. That's receptive aphasia. If I read a joke, I sometimes can understand it. But, thank God, I can understand what's funny inside me, and pass it on to others. To me, an IQ test in itself is funny.

I, who have a Ph.D. in theology, who can write books competently, find joy and laughter in translating Babel.

People with aphasia seldom mention to others what they've learned. But many fascinating people made it, translating the return to "normal" life. I, who love language skills and felt prisoned by aphasia, saw a list of famous people who had the disease. I got hope seeing Winston Churchill on the list. He liked crossword puzzles too. So . . . maybe I'll get back to the Sunday *Times* in the years ahead.

But deeper yet is my belief in God. With Him I have learned that in myself I am nothing. Language skills are nothing important at all. I had been "free." I had given my freedom to God, given myself back to the Lord to let Him do whatever He wants done. I am now very rich indeed.

And to understand that, you must realize what I was like in the summer of 1972.

# CRY BABEL

## CHAPTER ONE

Let's set the stage, that June.

Pick a sticky, hot night. I was sitting in the kitchen typing my thesis for my dissertation, due imminently at Fordham. During the day in New York, I was typing it and getting it Xeroxed, and coming home and typing at night. I lived on iced coffee. I reached into the refrigerator for more ice. There was no ice. The refrigerator had died.

So what would you do? Wipe your tears, make a joke, and get back to work. That June, everybody in the family was running around in circles. The living-room floors were being refinished, and the walls were being painted downstairs. The tent was ordered for the outside reception for the wedding of one of our sons. Their friends were working, fixing up the house, and various graduations were included. My study, as usual, was a mess. Termites had decided to break through the concrete into the study. Wings added to the horror of the house. Twenty good years, and then what?

Pay the exterminator, get the stink out, vacuum it, and some other time it would be painted. Meanwhile get back to the ordering of the buffet for the wedding, and buy a dress, and finish that thesis. The study was closed. I had as a professor graded the spring semester, but the papers and reports were unfiled. So by now you know what I was like: an overdoer, overachiever, and never neat, but interesting and never a bore. O.K.?

Also to set the stage, I introduce the family. It's always

difficult to write about a family, since private life is sacred. To help others understand aphasia, I must introduce them as they were in the summer of '72.

I was married to Martin Armstrong, a handsome lawyer. We had seven children, born in ten years, seven wonderful, fascinating people. With pride I name them to you: Marty, Michael, Cathy, Fulton, Caedmon, Clare, and Paul. Three were married, and the youngest was in junior high school. There were two grandchildren.

I am, and you would expect, a Catholic, a convert, baptized when I was twenty-one. Before joining the Church I had learned almost everything wrong with the Catholic Church and joyfully accepted it. With faith I committed myself to the holy, catholic, apostolic Church. More than anything in my whole life is my belief in the Trinity: the Father, the Son, and the Holy Spirit. I had fallen in love with God. Being totally imperfect, I gave my life to working, praying, studying, learning, cleaning, fixing, and trying to help others.

For various reasons, I had decided I had to become a theologian. That sounds like a show-off, and perhaps it was. But, from a woman's point of view, it was very difficult to stand forth and argue your belief with people who believe only priests know what's true. When Vatican II occurred, it became possible to be given a degree in theology.

Coming from a family of writers, I had learned my trade. I would never be a great writer, but competent at non-fiction, having a light touch with children's books and magazine articles and a dream of growing better at fiction. To learn the style of a dissertation is hard work. I had hated it. It took me four years to learn that game (using the *ibids.* contained in footnotes I had hated) and it was a style I became good at. Footnotes marched in my head. Then I found it difficult to write simply, in the normal swing.

"Stop being a theologian now. You made your point. Now get going and be you again." John Delaney, my kind editor, knew I owed him a book. "Drop the jargon. Get back to the typewriter. If you're rusty, as you are, write on anything from the refrigerator to the weeds outside. Your family taught you how to sit on your buttocks and sweat for hours daily. You'll get so bored writing about weeds, you'll get a new book going."

So, as July arrived, I would write on anything, and end up with footnotes and stodgy nonsense and throw the papers away.

Like any writer, I would stop and clean the study again, and look in the folders. I ended up opening my scrapbooks. I found a very old one with a childhood numerology chart stuck in a large envelope. Reading it was like having my fortune told, from 1926. Page by page, almost everything came true. I got up to my forty-fifth year and chuckled. The numerology writer had said that I would have a new title in my job. That was true. I was a wife, a mother, a grandma, and now, Dr. April Armstrong. I turned the page. There was nothing more. Nothing more about life.

I put that away quickly and went back to the typewriter. Delaney and I had agreed on modern mysticism. I began planning our synopsis.

But, afternoons, I sat in the shade outside with iced coffee, and loafed, and thought, and meditated. The four things always go together.

For an unknown reason, I had a strange feeling. Martin and I were planning to go to the lawyers' convention in San Francisco in August. Never before had I been nervous about going by airplane. I had always wanted to see San Francisco. Why, then?

Privately, there were some marital problems—at least on my side. In many ways, though we loved each other, we saw the world differently—everything from family quarrels to politics. But that wasn't unusual.

I sat next to the unweeded garden and meditated. Meditation was part of my life, even before the name Transcendental Meditation became the rage. Whom have I learned it from? From many people: from the Scriptures, from St. Teresa of Ávila, from biofeedback, from Jung, from Zen. You name it. Whether you agree or not, understand the way I was growing. Basically it was simple: You need to recognize yourself. You must be aware of many of your own parts and free yourself with openness. This means feeling your body, your mind, your unconscious level, and your spiritual level. Then, by will, you are free to be ready to grow. Unfortunately, some people emphasize certain aspects and levels over others. In meditating, one must be willing to admit one's human physical part, and know oneself well.

To meditate, one must begin with the body. And sitting in the shade, I kept feeling that something in my body was warning me. But, being no expert on my body, I could not understand the warning.

I phoned for an appointment to see my doctor, John Nagle, and have a good checkup. From my heart to my allergies I felt in good shape.

Yet, meditating, I sensed that I was physically ill.

Dr. Nagle was then on vacation, so I went to the one filling in for him. He admitted that I needed more allergy pills (the humidity of the summer, and the pollen was high). My diet was good. But perhaps, he said, you are just psychologically in need of a vacation. He was also a prayerful man. He said I would be able to go to San Francisco for the convention and return. Then my regular doctor would be back, and if I was still worried about my health, I could get some more checks done.

How beautiful San Francisco was! Particularly I loved the cathedral, the running water of the baptismal font, the music, the reverence for Our Lady of Guadalupe. At St. Mary's Cathedral, with the stained-glass windows of the elements of air, fire, water, and earth, I felt unafraid. The words of Our Lady of Guadalupe said: "Am I not your mother? Am I not life and health? Have I not placed you on my lap and made you my responsibility?" I bought a card and mailed it to the prayerful doctor.

I returned home unafraid.

Summer was almost over. Two children were about to go away to school: one to college, the other to boarding school. There were name tags to be sewed on, clothes to be bought, footlockers to be filled. But difficult problems continued between Martin and me. For the first time, we mentioned divorce. Or at least I did.

The house was tense. Dinner was terribly cool. I, who was usually looking for a reconciliation, was low, but different. I was sad, but not scared.

In our house, it was a special outing for the younger kids to drive over to Jones Beach to mark the end of summer. We had already planned it for Monday. I told Clare and Paul we would go.

Before going to sleep I prayed as usual. It was St. Augustine's Day, and he's a guy I had really come to understand well. It is necessary to be careful of truth, like Augustine, understand it well as you meditate, and then use your will to leap over to belief.

There was a prayer of St. Ignatius I had read many times. Truthfully, I would read it and not say it. It was in my breviary, and I read it that night. I realized it was time to make a decision. There were always reservations in myself, things I loved by myself, things I couldn't let go. Most of all, truthfully,

I knew that I felt too important. I had not yet given my freedom totally to God.

But, that night, I read it and meant it—an offering of myself.

Read it very carefully and understand it. It is a scary thing to say:

> Take, O Lord, and receive
>> my entire liberty,
>> my memory,
>> my understanding,
>> and my whole will.
>
> All that I am and all that I possess, You have
>> given to me.
>
> I surrender it all to you to be disposed of
>> according to Your will.
>
> Give me only Your love and Your grace.
>
> With these I will be rich enough, and will
>> desire nothing more.

I put the card next to my bed and fell asleep. Monday morning I had coffee, and since the children weren't awake, I decided to go back to bed to rest instead of rushing off to Jones Beach. Thank God!

I went back to my bedroom. And very slowly I fell to the floor.

Without yet knowing it, I was very rich.

Like it or not, I had dropped into the hand of God, the living God. If He wanted me to be handicapped, burdened with aphasia, and unable to be useful to others, that was His problem, and His use.

I was rich.

And, of course, being rich can also cause a lot of problems.

## CHAPTER TWO

What does it feel like when your brain gets undone?

Picture it this way. You are the person who bought a ticket and went into the theater. The lights go down. The movie begins. You begin to get involved in the story, halfway interested and halfway thinking it unreal. Then, suddenly, you see yourself in this strange film. You find yourself there as the star. Your mind begins to feel that you are split in two. But there is no time to interrupt, because you feel you have to pay strict attention. There is you the watcher, and there is you the actor, and both parts of you keep wondering about the producer of this film. The punk director surely loved fantasy sequences, Daliesque lights, and slow-motion shots. Suddenly the reel in the film apparently breaks. The lights go up. You shake your head. You turn to your family beside you. They look annoyed. No one seems to know what to say. The lights go down again. The movie continues, and you see yourself in that dream and you see your family in the movie. You put your hand onto their real hands in the dark, and there is no response. And in the movie they are not holding your hand.

Oh, my God—a dream upon a dream, nightmare upon nightmare. And no way out of this film.

Noise. Confusion. Babel.

Monday, August 28, 1972.

[To understand the real sequence, one need only remember that though I was very sick, no one could see anything wrong with me. No blood showing, no obvious stroke.]

I feel myself crumbling, in slow motion, to the green-blue rug. There is time to notice that darn' rug. I still haven't shampooed the rug. I will lie on it. I wonder if it smells doggy.

I want to get into bed. I wonder how to get there. Maybe I fainted. I've never fainted before. Clare [daughter]? I must be sick. I sort of push over to the bed. There is pain—but where is it? Not hard pain, just . . . I'm tired, too tired. Bed . . .

God, I'm cold.

"It's warm out," says Clare. She's using the phone in my bedroom and she's talking to the nurse. I don't want to talk to the doctor. I hate the world, and I hate you calling the doctor. Get the hell out of here. I'm sorry, gee I'm sorry. I guess we can't go to Jones Beach. I'm yelling. I'm screaming.

"Get out of here!"

I can hear myself shouting, and wonder why. . . .

Clare. Paul [son].

"You've got to go to the doctor."

O.K., you pain, Clare. So you went downstairs and called the nurse again? But Dad said Fulton [son] can't drive the car because of the fight. I don't feel like driving.

Terrible headache. I cry. Fulton can drive me to the doctor's office.

"O.K., but I've got a lot of things to do to get ready for Georgetown. If I can't drive, I'll have to go with my friends."

Use my car.

I put on clothes and remember we were having a family fight last night. I forgot. So who cares! But see everyone is uptight.

"Need help getting dressed, Mom? Don't just sit there."

Putting on clothes that are far away, even in my hands. Really as though my body and my clothes are disjointed. My hands move my clothes over my body, but I'm not sure that these are my hands doing it. I am getting dressed while I stand aside from myself and watch.

Everything is so far away.

The stairs from the second floor to the first floor are huge.

[Partway down the stairs, my brain sent a flashback. When I was eleven years old I nearly died with a disease called tularemia. When I was recuperating, I was very weak and was not allowed to walk down the stairs at first. I had to push my way down the stairs sitting-sliding, one step at a time.]

My God, I've got tularemia again. That's why I should tell the doctor. Something awful is going on. I'll sit-slide down. I'm scared.

"Tularemia!" I cry, and the pain is great. "Why can't you understand?"

I get to the living-room chair and rest. I am using my strength to stop crying and to be in charge.

"Fulton, I have to go slowly. I can't go quickly."

The car is nine miles away. . . .

I wake. I guess I slept in the car. Here are the stairs to Dr. Nagle's office. There are a few steps and about ten yards to the office. It is so far away. I start to sit in a chair. The nurse says I must go downstairs to the lab. I can't. I can't.

"Mom."

I will, of course. I'm teary and I hold my head.

[Time is elastic. I would have sworn it took me an hour to go up and down the stairs and into various rooms. By other people's watches it took about five minutes. I would have sworn I'd fallen asleep, wakened, and moved forward very slowly. But anyone watching me knew I didn't fall asleep and that I handled things well.]

Geesus! I'm going blind. The blind feeling is on me. Each step is a steep cliff. Is it being blind, or is it a dream, or did the eye sockets get swollen? A bigger step, an abyss. One abyss after another. Go down some stairs and into the lab.

"Hi! Glad it's someone I know." That's me.

"You know me well."

I know she thinks I'm kooky. I pull myself together, twirling in my head. "Moving must make me dizzy."

"O.K. You go on back to Nagle's office."

I swallow tears and start to go. Stiff climb—each step so far away. On the ground floor and I insist I will not go any farther. I'm tired. I'm very tired. Fulton, damn it, I will not go up to the office. Take me home.

"O.K., O.K. Don't make so much noise."

"I think I have the flu. I'm mad."


[Remember, deep illness doesn't occur politely; it doesn't occur in a vacuum. Many patients, with everything from gall-bladder conditions to strokes, were also under high levels of stress. These stresses, with guilt among the worst of them, stay with the patient and family.

[If I were Martin, I might have done the same thing: got angry at the doctor, wondering how sick I really was.]

You've been talking to me, Martin, but I guess I was asleep.

"Do you want something to eat?"

"No!"

I've been in the bathroom throwing up. No, I don't have a fever. I'm just sick. Don't get angry at the doctor.

"I called Nagle and he won't come to our house. He said we should bring you to the emergency room. I'm furious at him."

I haven't got strength for a fight.

"What a lousy doctor! I'm not going to take you to the emergency room."

Impasse. Anger from yesterday. I go back and throw up. I

won't go to any doctor either. I have flu and I have tularemia
and I'm tired.

"Can I have some ginger ale?" The poor kids are making a
lousy dinner.

Tuesday.

Oh, no—I'm telling you: I'm having another baby.

No. No baby.

Why? Had them all.

I'm almost awake. Nausea usually meant being pregnant.
But now I'm just nauseated.

"Mike [son], I don't want to go to the doctor."

"I'll get you there, Mom. You've got to go. Clare called me.
And look, Fulton and me just picked you up from the floor.
You can't do that!"

I look at Clare and I am scared. Very scared. I'd better get
my wits together.

"Clare, help me."

[She changed and dressed me while I kept rattling on about
how my mother told me to put on good clothes in case you end
up in an accident. I blacked out a number of times. I became
aware that I was in Dr. Nagle's office.]

I'm glad I like you. I'm not sure what's the matter. I'm too
tired to ask why.

[By the time I got to St. Joseph's Hospital, I was making no
sense. Mike called Dad in New York to tell him, and went
home to bring Clare to me.]

Awful dark here. Why so many tests?

[Martin runs in.] He's scared and I'm scared.

"Hi!" I'm proud of saying it out loud. "Hi. It's not tularemia." Why the hell am I saying that? Something is wrong. I'm
going to sleep. Now.

Larger room. Still St. Joseph's Hospital. How did I get here? Sit up. See Ruth Schmidt and Celine Heath. Old friends, but also nurses. Just sitting there looking at me. What are they here for?

I look at them and that frightens me. I look at the window, early morning. Oh, yeah, I remember. No one knows what's wrong with me. I look at them with a phony smile so they won't be worried.

My head hurts, headache and severe pain in my neck and legs. They help me lie back. You're not working nurses for me today, are you? Just visiting?

"Just came to see you. Rest."

Oblivion is nice.


[At times I seemed quite normal. I would phone my kids. My daughters-in-law were helping Clare to get the last things needed for boarding school. My closest friends, Jo and Bill Moran, who had been visiting with us all a few days ago, called from Hazleton. I talked coherently, about pain and tests. But a few minutes later I called my son Marty, and his wife, Kathy, and talked like a drunken bum, quite incoherent.

[Martin was back and forth, working, talking with the doctors, and doing the million jobs needed for the kids returning to school. I kept asking why the children didn't visit. They weren't allowed to. The tests were often, thank God, leaving me in oblivion.]

I wake up. I see Father Watts sitting in a chair beside me. I push myself up. He says I mustn't. He's worried, because I should lie still.

"I want to go to confession. So you don't have a stole? Who cares? I have to do this because it takes all the strength I've got."

Two things wrong I did, Father. I'm sorry. I don't remember the words. I feel dizzy. Words don't matter.

Help me lie down.

Whoopee! That's done. All set. I'm free to go.

[Brother X. Sabrini, a good, kind man, of the Third Order of St. Francis, sneaked Clare and Fulton into my hospital room in the early morning. Fulton was going to Georgetown, Clare to Westover.]

I'm crying. I'm furious. I hate you all because I cannot go. Dad was taking you to Georgetown and he's not going to do it. And I wanted to go to Westover with you, my alma mater. I'm stuck here.

"Shh. The nurses will throw us out!"

A kiss. A blessing. A goddam good-by.

I don't know why. I don't know. I don't know.

[Why did this scene occur? It would have been sweet to have a life-and-death "farewell" speech. But it didn't. Part of that was aphasia, words and emotions off kilter. But part of it was a communication gap in the family—a very common complaint to all families hit with deep illness.

[Rather than worry the children, particularly for those who were entering a situation of new schools, Martin told them I was just having light tests done. He did not tell them how serious things were. With real conviction, he felt he had to seem calm in order to help them. He himself was fantastically scared.

[But, looking back on it, I beg others to believe in a family's need to know the whole truth, with no reservations. Children of *any* age find security in knowing that they are in on it. Truth is actually more kind than putting up a front. To spell out one's own fear is showing true love. If you don't know what may happen, talk it out.

[When I said good-by to Clare and Fulton, I did not know that they did not know how scared I was. I was angry that they did not share my known fear. They thought I was sarcas-

tic, teary, and not being myself. It would take more than a
year for that communication gap to be healed.

[Many years ago, Martin and I had made a pact that we
would pull no punches in illness. The tests completed, Martin
had to tell what was in store. We held hands, and kissed. We'd
have to wait and see and pray.]

I want to die. I'm dying to die. Funny; true.

The Lord will take care of me. Oh, yeah? I'd rather die. I
will die. God damn it.

I feel safe. In.

I feel terrified. Screaming! Out.

Who's screaming? Oh, my God. That's me screaming. Yup!
Animal me. Part of my mind actually is shaking my head, saying to myself . . . April, you're really crazy.

God damn it, don't give me another shot. . . .

"I want to die, Tony [my brother]. Dying is easier than living. I could go up to heaven and still be me. But to be a vegetable and not to be myself?"

"Are you scared, April?"

"Sometimes. I hear myself screaming and I disagree with
what I scream at. Hold my hand. I'm in two pieces."

I gotta go to the bathroom. How ya get over the rail? I'll
mess the place. My Mummy'll be back soon.

[I was sure I was in Boston Hospital, eleven years old, with
tularemia. I climbed over the rail and fell on the floor. I partly
knew I was forty-five and partly kept talking about playing a
game like Scrabble, thirty-four years ago. I was terrified. I
knew my mother was long dead, but another piece of my
memory was reminding me that one cannot go to the bathroom
in the bed.

[The second time I crawled out to the bathroom and fell, I
had to be restrained. My mind was split into pieces.

[The hemorrhage continued. The artery on the left side of my brain was deeply in spasm. Martin made the correct decision to bring me by ambulance to New York Hospital. With Martin's sister, Mary, and our close friend Dr. Al Dunn, radiology specialist, Martin believed the best neurosurgeon for me was Bronson Ray. The odds were against me. There was no guarantee, even on moving me. An operation was out of the question until the spasm relaxed. Relax? Typical of me! Typical of me, trying to run my own show.

[Poor Martin! I understood his decision, and agreed. He was holding my hand, and we would face whatever was ahead. What can a husband and wife say? I love you and you love me. God help us.

[In times of stress, coincidences are gorgeous. For twenty years, every child on our block knew and loved Gus the mailman. Gus was also a volunteer fireman. Who can be afraid of traveling in that ambulance with Gus? Not me! A man who is close to the Lord?

[The nurses in the neurosurgery wing of New York Hospital were superwomen. Two years later, I was able to find several of them and thank them, separately. They had a special touch, were hard-working, competent, but beyond that, giving that special gift of hope, personal awareness, and security. A word, a belief in the future—these are the gifts to hold us when we cannot see the next five minutes, let alone the future. My nurses at New York Hospital were holding my rope of life, which seemed to me to be a high cliff, so foggy that one cannot see the top . . . or the bottom.

[Daily, Martin would take the train to New York, to work, to visit me, and take the train home to Stamford to be with young Paul, cook and bottle washer. In many ways, my time was easier than Martin's. The worry, the decisions, the fear are worse for the well than for the sick. The job of the sick is to accept and wait, like it or not.

[At the time, only my closest relatives were allowed to visit me. My brother, Tony, and his wife, Noel. Martin's sister, Mary. And Father Peter Mongiano, I.M.C. Father Peter, busy with his own mission work in New Jersey, would drive to Stamford to spend a few nights with young Paul, then visit New York Hospital.

[Suspended time . . . the time of waiting, before the decision for the operation. Two weeks or so, suspended.

[I was lucky. Those visiting with me were giving all their energy to me. Quite often, I was, as one would say, "out cold." But I could understand half of what was going on, even when apparently asleep. You never know! I tell you: the soul is awake even if the body is asleep.

[Talk to the sleeping patient: to him, not about him. Dignity and reverence are needed for all people, and especially for those too ill to communicate. Where are the body and soul? I had at times heard Martin talking out loud, crying, assured that I was "out." I could not reach him, and I felt so sorry for him. I could not answer back.

[I'm not a teacher of psychology. But, from my way of seeing it, I found at least three levels of consciousness. First, the level of talking, on which what one says reaches the conscious level of one who understands. Second, the level of physical reaction, the guts. Third, the level of the spirit.

[Let's see if you can see through my focus.]

[Broken conscious level]

Martin, my darling. Thank God for music. He has hung my FM radio over my bed. Another battery. Poor you. But without music what would I do? You look tired, Martin.

I don't want to eat. O.K., I'll eat.

I never get to see my doctors. I'm always asleep when they come.

[A few moments clearly seen.] Sure, I'll be all right. Father
Peter, sing a song with me. Bum lah da bum bum, bum bum!
What fun! Martin, you do a vaudeville dance. God, how lovely
you are, and Peter, and I know all three of us are walking on
eggs.

[Blackout]

Tony . . . you laugh . . . you laugh well. Aren't we lucky
that we like each other. Laughter feels great, and hurts!
Brother and sister, we end up hysterically laughing when the
stress is too much. . . .

But, Tony, I may not make it, right? Dr. Ray called you,
didn't he?

[I looked at Tony and understood. Dr. Ray was to operate
on me soon. And I might end up as a vegetable. Was it ESP?
Tony did not tell me that at the time. But somehow I knew
that my brother was aware. I did not cry until he left. And
then I screamed and screamed and screamed. Release of
horror.]

Father Freddie? How did you get here?

[Father Freddie, a priest from Bombay, studying new
methods for helping the deaf and mute, came to bring the
Anointing of the Sick. Two women I did not know were
there. Everyone agreed that I was deeply asleep. My eyes were
closed.

[Yet I saw the whole scene.

[I began thinking that one ought to make notes, to prove the
levels of communication, so that others can study it. But I
could not move. It might take years before I could write it
down.

[It would take me two years to prove my point. At a church
in Stamford I saw a woman, and remember her as the one on

the right in the hospital room where I was asleep, eyes closed. She remembered me. Proof, to me, that one can see without seeing.]

[The level of the physical body, disjointed . . .]

Nice nurses. You are taking me where? [The nurses tell me the orderlies will bring me to a place for tests.] Listen, men, what are you doing? You're pushing me along, and talking over me as though I don't exist.

Don't say: Lie still. You don't hear me because what I said sounds crazy. Goddam it.

I am alone.

Bees!! Oh-hhh, be-e-e-e-s. All over me. Around me. Spiders that bite. Yah-h-h-h!

Monkeys sit on nothing.

Jackals and buzzards, waiting. . . .

And the damn' pain!

I cry all the way back to my hospital room. Whimpering, and it sounds stupid of me but I can't stop. I am so scared. "They" might be there again.

Oh, nurse. You hug me. Oh, God, you hug me like a child and I need you. You're telling me what was going on. You tell me again and again, and rock me.

They are doing something more.

I am in the desert, buried in the sand up to my neck. Only my head is free—what a way to get tests!

Only my head. Now they are dropping honey all over my face. Black ants, tremendous black ants, are going to eat me alive. I cannot move. I'm stuck under the heavy sand. I wish I could die. I— I— I— I—

Will anyone rescue me?

[That nightmare was the worst. It was so awful that I could

not permit myself to remember it until February 1976. The mind sometimes swallows fear and sticks it deep in the unconscious: amnesia. Three and a half years after the operation, I was writing a chapter of this book. My unconscious allowed me to write about the ants in the desert. I could not spell the word "ants." I left my study, and began crying, looking in the dictionary for the way to spell "ants."

[I was very distraught. I remembered the dream. But I remembered a movie I had seen years before. The brain put the two pieces together. In the hospital, unaware of what the tests were for, the body used the dream to explain the physical anguish and fear of the tests.

[With joy I could let the pus of the unconscious escape, and spit out the horror of not knowing what was going on!

[How many other aphasics have bad dreams? And fear that cannot be thrown out without help? Part of the dreams is physical disjointed memories. And part of them is anger and frustration bottled up in aphasia.]

[Two levels, then: the conscious and the physical. And the third level is the spiritual level.

[Strange, how nervous it is to mention the sacred core of one's life to others. To mention God?]

You are there. "You walk with me and You talk with me. . . ." I sing it with You, Lord. But—my God—it is not a song. It is real. You are there.

[Awe. Awe that runs through one's body and soul. A different kind of fear. In English we use one word, "fear," for two totally different meanings. Fear of horror is quite different from fear of God. The fear of awe and the fear of a kiss exist in the "fear of the Lord."]

Oh, my God.

[There is no word to express the feeling, the presence, of God. Time is gone. It was different from the first two levels. It was so *sweet*, the ecstasy so constant—with no beginning and no end—that it was more alive than anything I had dreamed.]

No one would ever believe me.

People would laugh at it—or would they?

"No eye has ever seen. . . ."

Oh, Jesus.

He laughs gently, and seems to sit me down beside Him.

"See!" It is His voice.

I see Jesus with me, and ahead the Trinity. No words. Words without words. Sound, spiral, music without music.

Three in one. One in three. Oh, my God!

"April, remember it. Remember it. Remember it."

I cannot hear the words. I cannot hear what they're saying.

He laughs, so genially. "You think these are just words?"

I feel so safe that I can talk with Him. A child, safe.

"Can I stay here?"

"No, April. You must go back."

The seeing of the Trinity is gone. I look at Jesus and He nods with a smile again.

"You wonder why I am here with you, and there with the Trinity?"

"Yes."

You know, no one will believe what is going on? That's blasphemy for me to write this down. . . .

"Where are you? With Me. Where am I? With you. Where were you before? Here. Where will you be? Here. I Am."

Without words, I understood what was necessary:

I am a nothing, and Jesus holds me. He's human. He is also divine. He is God, God, God. He is around me, in me, through me. He is in you, too. If you wish to, and fall into Him, you are at once nothing and everything.

[Partly, I kept hoping the "dreams" would disappear. They would not. Nor are they a demented memory scale. I kept hoping that I could keep it private. I could not.

[After five years, quite back in the stream of modern life, I am aware that to write of this is difficult, publicly. I who hate super-pious nonsense, of which there is a lot, wish to hell I didn't have to write it.]

"Because so many other people know the same thing and don't communicate to the world. It's your job."

"No one will believe me."

"So?" said Jesus.

"Can I make it anonymous?"

"You will be a child."

"Walk with Me."

With His hand in mine, I had been beholding the Three-in-One. Suddenly we were in it. Not long. This is not sound, music, words. This is—

Only a moment. A spiral Three-One, One-in-Three. . . .

He put me back, not as Son but as Jesus watching.

"You must hold on. Mary will help you remember. Ask her. You are going to forget for a while. But, the important things, she will hold for you."

"Can't I die? Now?"

"No, dear. You have a job to do here for a while."

"When will I go back?"

"The time will come when the end is done. Open the front door and you will see Me quite differently. You will be old then, and you will see Me."

Jesus, you know me. I am a mess. I even use Your word for everything from anger to joking. A good saint has learned how to behave. This is unreal.

"This is ultimately real," said Jesus.

"Your love for me, Jesus—I believe Your love, but it seems unreal when I think on it."

"Hush."

"Jesus, if You are Jesus, how can You—"

I was too scared to say what I was thinking. I could accept Jesus as my Brother and my King but—as a symbol, as an awesome love. But a woman who is less than perfect, cross, fat —you name it—one would have to think herself in need of psychological help. It used to distress me when I read of mystics who used sexual words for the love of God. Their writings of sugar sweetness used to make me want to vomit. My idea of God, and theirs, were quite different.

"You're just being you, April. And I am telling you to relax and let Me run you."

"May I see Dad and Mother?"

"They are with you."

"Is the time going on? I mean, Teilhard said the end of life of the world is going on forever?"

"He was right on so much, dear. But the end is much closer. On this he was wrong, of course. . . . April, you can't ask so many questions. Remember. All you need to know is that the Church is not just the Vatican, nor the Pope. The Church is in Me. The time will be coming, when this Pope has died, and the schism will rock the boat of Peter. There will be some on one side and some on the other. The conclave will not agree. You will feel closer to the Anglican rite, and the priests will be confused. The Eucharist is to be hidden in people's houses, in homes. No one will be sure whose Eucharist is real. The *anawim*, the laymen, will live through it. Judge not lest you be judged."

Silence.

## CHAPTER THREE

I woke, and remembered last night. "It's over, darling. You're all right. All you have to do is get strong again," Martin had said. Alleluia. Thank God. Thank You, Jesus. I felt good. I saw the nurse and smiled.

"Damn I hell hell damn shit?"

The inflection was mine, polite, but weak and childlike. The nurse was answering, but I broke in.

"God damn it?"

I was listening to my own sound.

Maybe there's a bad connection, I thought. No. There couldn't be a bad connection, because I'm not talking over the phone. I coughed.

"Bullshit?"

I thought I heard what I said.

The nurse was talking to me. I strained to listen to her voice.

"Here's your breakfast coming, April. You're talking, and that's great. But don't get scared. Your words may frighten you, but relax. It will all work out in the end."

She helped me. "Here's your pillow. Push yourself up a bit." As she let me sip orange juice, she carefully told me a bit about aphasia.

"Inside, on the left side of the brain, there is a strange map, where all obscenity is located. Don't worry about it so much. You cannot control it at all. Quite soon it will disappear again."

"Crap?" As nearly as I understood it, I was saying *What?*

The nurse told me again about the brain, and also told me

how wonderful I am, and how lucky I am because my vocal cords are working well.

I kept talking to her. She kept assuring me, and letting me swallow some breakfast. I talked constantly, hoping she knew my language. Like some people in foreign lands, I talked louder and slower. It didn't work. The louder I spoke, the more foul language I heard coming from me.

"You'll feel better not talking so much. We don't mind, because we know your problem, and we know what a great gal you really are. Our job is to make it easier for you. In a few days the real bad words will recede. And we will smile at you when the good words appear."

"Oh, damn it to hell!" Which meant exactly that. I closed my eyes and wondered when the nightmare would go away. It didn't. I thought back. Last night, after the recovery room, Martin had been beside me, holding my head and talking. I had not talked much, being drowsy. But with love, he promised me, everything would work out, and he would take care of me.

So I was sure that at least Martin would talk English with me. But when he came, and I talked to him, I could hear the strange language that came from me.

"Lady, damn it to hell?" Which meant, *Martin, what's going on?*"

He said, "You're having breakfast!"

Babel! Babel was true.

"Lady?" I asked.

"My name's Martin."

I agreed. "Lady!" *Martin* is the word. But the brain sent out *Lady*.

Oh, my God. I'm in another warp level. Jonathan Swift wrote a story about living in another world.

Tears fell near my nose. What I meant to say was, "Will it

get better? They said I wouldn't feel like that always! I'm not crazy, am I?"

"April, I know, and the nurses know too. It's all right!"

I wanted to close my mouth and say nothing. But I wanted to talk. Anathema words, uncharitable words, foul oaths, slang expressions, these I had. Kind words, good words? Practically gone.

"Try 'euphemism.'" Martin at least made me laugh.

Mortification, God.

I wanted to disappear.

"You have a big day ahead. Dr. Ray said you have to get out of bed and sit in a wheelchair, to move a bit. You have been lying down for almost a month. You're awfully weak."

I didn't want to.

"Noel is coming. And Pat Benzmiller." He watched to see if I could remember them. I nodded.

Sure enough, as Martin went to work, I ended up in a wheelchair, next to the window to see the world outside. Many people knew I loved to collect frogs, so frogs started appearing in my hospital room in various shapes and sizes. Pat gave me a small stuffed frog, and Mary, Martin's sister, gave me two. One was small enough for me to hold in my hand. It kept me company. Noel gave me a ride down the corridor. The noise of people talking was incredible. Much later, I would realize that this noise level is normal for aphasics. But, at the time, I listened to normal people taking for granted the hundred sounds of life: a shoe sound, a sole sound, a ripped paper, a cough. When you do not know what these things are for, you quickly tire.

I fell asleep holding my frog.

Jesus was next to me. I bit my hands and didn't know what to say.

"You're angry, April. Good." He seemed to change and grow, and then picked me up into His huge hands. "When you're angry, let the truth come out. You're furious at Me."

"No . . . but—"

"Well?"

"Yes."

"You are as a child. A strange child, but My child. Trust Me." The trust filled me, and I snuggled in His arm.

"There, there," He said, and walked down by the sea and let me feel the breeze. "There is no pretense, no dissembling, no sham. You cannot tell a lie now even if you wanted to. You are free. You cannot hide from Me, and I love you. The trouble is that most people are not free. They put up false images between themselves and Me. I see them, but they don't see Me."

I kept quiet.

"Tell Me what you really think."

"Why did You do this to me? I'm living a nightmare." I wondered if He would be angry with me for saying the truth.

"You're not ready for really understanding all of it. But let's say I want you to learn how to translate Babel. Now sleep for a while."

I felt safe with Him.

But I would wake with terror.

I could not stand to be alone, I who loved silence. The fear was constant when I was awake and alone. I slept little.

Martin, the family, and nurses moved me to a larger room with other patients, but fear grew there with the unknown. Noise, people I could not see clearly, was worse. Martin had me brought back to my original room, and set up a routine so I'd know what was going on.

During the early morning, a wonderful close friend from Stamford, Mary Ball, would drive down to the city to stay with me. She, who hated driving in traffic, left her four teen-agers, brought her thermos and lunch, and spent the whole day with me. Mary Ball would leave at four, and in half an hour Martin would come, smiling. His sister, Mary Armstrong, or Tony would arrive too. Then Martin would take the train home to be with Paul and the house, and I would be alone and scared. The nurses would move me out into the corridor so I could watch the people going by. And soon my night nurse would arrive.

Unfortunately I can't find her name, but I bless her often. A dignified, beautiful black woman, a woman of true charity. She had a way of knowing and translating what I was saying. We talked for hours.

She was unmarried, and I hoped she would become interested in the doctor from Nigeria who was spending a year interning in our country.

"Typical of a child, you are," the nurse chuckled. "You're trying to be a matchmaker?"

I would insist she should go to the lounge for coffee. And I would get angry, because the minute she crossed to the room opposite from mine, I found myself scared again.

"Why am I so scared, like a baby?"

She and the doctor sat next to me and explained.

"Surgery in the brain is much like a large earthquake. Tremors continue much longer than the operation. The stuff in your brain is much like jelly that has been put in a mixer. The brain reels. Remember what it feels like in an airplane, or a high elevator, or swimming under water? Sometimes it takes a couple of days to get the pressure out of your tubes. Well, with your brain it takes much longer. The brain doesn't give you pain. Instead, it hurts with *fear*."

I understood in simple language.

"*This* fear is a physical disorder that will pass. The other fear isn't in your system. You're a staunch and true gal. You've got a hard job ahead. You've got to work for getting well. You're going to physical therapy."

I was learning. But she knew I needed help. The second week, she fell in the street, but she came, limping with pain. It wasn't the money that brought her to work, but charity. I certainly needed her support.

Mary Ball wheeled me into the large therapy room with its old-fashioned floor, almost like a garret, filled with modern equipment. I met the therapists, who worked with a right mixture of loving gentleness and the stamina of sergeants.

I saw the parallel bars.

"We're going to help you to stand and hold on. Look at the mirror as you hold on."

Quickly I looked at the large mirror. And saw myself.

Oh, my God!

I opened my eyes, and psychologically blanked it out.

I looked at the mirror, and I saw the stair behind me, and Mary Ball, and the therapist. But I did not see me.

It was at least four minutes before I could even remember how I reacted.

"You turned sideways and looked at me. You looked like you were going to faint. Then you shook your head and looked in the mirror and looked happy," said Mary. "I asked you later, but you had no memory of anything about the mirror at all, until winter came."

What one cannot emotionally handle, one dismisses into the unconscious. I could not accept the image of myself that September. I could use the big mirror to walk with, I could see the image of the parallel bars. I could see others beside me. But I couldn't stand the sight of myself.

At least for women, the image of the face is important. In surgery, the left side of my head was shaven. The hair on the right side was filthy, long and scrawny, and ugly. What woman could look at that unkempt hair, that half-bald, half-crazy wife?

God love Mary Ball. Back in my room, she got the right permission from the doctors and nurses, and, by hook or by crook, she washed my hair in the sink.

[The amnesia lasted about four months. At home, my friend and beautician, Jo Novaral, came and gave me a crew cut. I would sit near a large window in our downstairs playroom in the evening and watch the reflection in the glass. I could see Martin, my little dog, Poltergeist, family, and friends. But there was no reflection of me. Then, one night, in the kitchen I looked at a dining-room window and recognized myself!

["Martin! Look! Oh, wow!" I ran to the bathroom mirror. He came running.

["Oscar Wilde! That's why I couldn't see me, Martin."

[Poor Martin. How could he understand what I was saying? But he kept writing it down for me, and slowly it made sense to doctors and families with aphasia. As an aphasia reporter, my language skills were off. My vocabulary was small. I could not formulate amnesia or the emotional trauma of a self-image. So my memory picked up from the storehouse a story written by Oscar Wilde. (There is, of course, a difference between his famous story and my memory of his story.) As I remembered it, Wilde told of a man who had a painting of himself. The man kept the painting in his attic, where no one would ever see it. The man stayed young and handsome, year after year. But the painting changed and aged, leaving every mark of evil and destruction. Only when the man died did his real face show how awful he was. The painting returned to being fresh and innocent.

[I got Martin to write down my notes. I was trying to explain the psychological image of aphasics. The doctors weren't deeply interested. I was. I knew that there would be years for me to be able to reread my Jung and relearn about myself. But at least I was on the track back to reality.

[More than anything, the handicapped and disabled need a good image of themselves. It takes gumption to look at a mirror image of oneself. Only love, and hope, from others can fill that hole.]

I understood that the way to get well, and go home to my own house, was to work at therapy. And therapy meant both physical and mental, including tests.

A table with colored wooden shapes was placed before me. Part of me cringed. Far, far away in my mind I knew there were symbolic IQ tests. But part of me always loved games, and simple colors delighted me.

Physical exercising was more difficult. The right side of my body was numb. Therapists exercised my hands, arms, and legs. When they moved me, I could be polite. But when they wanted me to do my share, I was downright nasty. I was rude, and I felt awfully sorry for myself, trying to hold on to the parallel bars and looking at my feet.

Then, as I kept talking loudly with my oaths, I became aware of a very young teen-ager next to me, doing her tasks. She was the most grotesque child I ever saw. She had no fingers, only stubs. Her eyes and her face dripped constantly with liquid. She had almost no skin. She looked like a peeled onion.

She was learning how to sew.

At a break from my exercising, the worker told me the girl had never lived anywhere else but in this hospital. The therapists, the nurses, the maids, and the elevator operators—these were her family.

Oh, poor child! Compared to her, I had no problem. I wouldn't black out my memory of her, but swallowed my self-pity and tried again.

On the sixth day my therapist told me the hardest test was ahead of me. But when I learned it, I'd be able to go home.

"April, you've been sitting, and standing. But fairly soon you've got to learn how to fall."

She reminded me as a mother that some babies learn how to stand up in the crib and scream because they don't know how to let go.

"Remember how you taught them to sit down? Remember as a mother teaching them trust, to be unafraid?"

But at forty-five years old?

"The soft mat on the floor is the same one you have been exercising on. You just have to—"

I shook my head.

The therapist said it wasn't time for that test yet. She wheeled me into other interesting rooms, to look at the kitchen, and the bathroom. I got to play games with blocks. But I knew that tomorrow, or the next day, I would have to learn how to fall. And thinking of it, I got teary, and exhausted. At the end of my appointment I fell asleep in the wheelchair on the way back to my room.

And, as usual, after napping I woke up with fear again. I saw Martin, and laughed. "Lady!"

Martin was bringing mail, flowers, and a new battery for the transistor radio.

"You're growing better! You're doing great! And they're going to take the catheter out tomorrow."

"Baby money?" *Money,* or *Mummy*—no one was sure which word it was. The inflection can mean anything at all. *Lady* meant only *Martin.*

"The catheter." He pointed.

I looked at this thing beside me.

"It's been with you wherever you've been. Now you won't need it."

I had never noticed it. It had no meaning for me.

In the morning the catheter was removed. My goodness, what a feeling! Any psychologist could understand the trauma in me. It was almost like having the umbilical cord cut, lost, separated. As an aphasic, far, far away in my brain I was fascinated with my texts on Freud. Until that moment, I had no memory of bedpans or bowel movements. The higher brain wondered what had gone on for a month. The baby level of my brain was having fun.

One level of me said silently: "Oh, euphemism! By God! I really am a baby all over, and I am mortified."

The second level was rewarded by doing my duty. And I was proud of myself. The door, of course, was open.

The first level began to realize my nightmares were true.

"It's a good sign, April. You have to stay in the hospital until you're able to handle all the bathroom facilities—and until you learn how to fall on the floor."

I wanted to go home.

"I love you," said Martin.

"You'll make it," said Mary Ball.

"You will," said Tony.

*I will do it. By God. I will do it.*

I couldn't let go.

They helped me to sit on the mat and taught me to lie down sideways.

"Hooray! You did well. Now sit up sideways again."

I managed it.

"Now we want you to pull yourself up while we hold you." I watched, and understood what they were saying. I also understood what I was afraid of, and what they were interested in. I put my left hand over my head and hoped they guessed my question.

"April!" said Mary Ball. "Your head will never break! Remember? The doctor showed it to you. You are very safe. Some people with bandages will bleed if they fall. But yours won't."

"Baby. Mummy."

Mary Ball turned to the therapist. "I think April wants to talk about why falling is necessary. She's a smart gal. But she knows her right hand won't move to catch her."

"Your right side will move, April. You are not paralyzed. You're just partly paralyzed. I believe that if you start to fall, your involuntary movements of the body will react. You will fall, but you will know how to fall."

"Money damn it?"

The therapist told me again with gestures. I laughed at Mary Ball and nodded with a *whew!* on the left side. It took time to override my dread. But finally I let go. The right side involuntarily reacted for the floor, the knees bent, the hands caught at the right time.

Happy tears.


Jesus was there with me.

I said to Him, "You're the only person I can communicate with totally."

"Yes."

I looked at Him and He laughed. "Talk out your feelings to Me. You think that's not fair, not being able to talk perfectly to others. But you don't want to mention it to Me!"

I felt ashamed.

"April, you said you gave yourself to Me. And now you still aren't ready to say your feeling out loud to Me. You're angry at Me. Then, say it. If you are a friend, you must tell the truth."

"Why did You do this to me? I'm terrified."

He hugged me. "No barriers. No pretending. God is not polite. God is not a thing, or a time. God is. So many people won't talk to God if they are going to the bathroom, or feeling angry, or shaking with frustration. God is in each person, but most people don't believe it. We exist everywhere."

"Believe in You. And so, O.K., I believe You picked the worst cross for me. No words, no books, no nothing." The moment I said it, I giggled and felt better.

But He shook His head. "You can't pretend to smile and laugh when you feel that way. That is unreal. In a way, you will find the paradox of your life now. But, for the moment, say the truth: you don't know how to say the mystery, but you're angry at Me. Don't be scared of that."

I had stopped smiling.

## CHAPTER FOUR

More than anything, I needed a friend.

Aphasics need a tremendous amount of help in the first few months. At that time we are mostly floating in space, feeling almost drunk, as though we are dancing on another planet and only occasionally touching base on this earth. Maudlin words swing through memory, trying to communicate to the normal world. Someone has to make decisions for the family, and their work is difficult and lonely.

Martin cared for me well. He understood that an aphasic needed one doctor to co-ordinate one's needs, keeping tabs on everything from prescriptions and blood-pressure tests to the nitty-gritty questions of allergies and constipation. (Constipation is not funny after a stroke!) With Dr. Nagle I felt safe.

Martin understood that one needs physical therapy for rehabilitation. He chose St. Joseph's Hospital, and with Dr. John Casey I felt safe. So, too, would I feel safe with Ben Cariri, a private speech pathologist.

Why do I use that word *safe* so often? With fear heavy on the brain, aphasics need to feel safe. They need to feel the goodness of their doctor and their teachers. Confidence in themselves is totally lost. Like children, they notice the empathy of others. I was lucky, for I had Martin, who was aware that I needed empathy and safety in my new role.

He also knew that I could not be left alone until the fear subsided and I could take care of myself. I didn't need a nurse. I needed a baby-sitter who was stimulating, knowledgeable, and likable. What I needed was a friend who believed in me. But who in the world would do that?

Martin pondered. Then he had the daring to ask Mary Ball.

What kind of person was she? She and her husband, Bud, had four children. As the youngsters grew into their teens, Mary and Bud volunteered to foster newborns waiting for adoption papers to be filed. During the day, wherever Mary went, little babies went too. In the evening Bud and the teenagers helped, taking love as part of life. Looking in their albums with pictures of thirty different babies, I had asked them only one question: Was it just luck that not one single infant screamed constantly? Was it luck that the babies learned swiftly how to sleep through the two o'clock bottle? Or was it love and security?

Bud and Mary had enough to do without helping me. But Bud and Mary answered immediately. "If April needs help, we'll bring the baby to her house every day. Somehow we'll manage."

And Mary stopped by to talk to me.

"Look. I don't know how to be a real nurse. But if you're not scared with me bumbling things around, and if you're not embarrassed with a friend, let's see how it works!"

Oh, boy, did I feel safe!

Martin would give me coffee before he left on the seven-thirty to New York. I had learned that I could not touch the stove. Just before eight, Paul left for school. And by eight-thirty Mary wheeled the baby carriage into my dining room and the day started.

"I'll turn on the shower for you, hon."

On my right hand I felt no difference. On my left hand I was learning the difference between hot and cold. But while I reacted with pain on the left, I had not learned which side the spigot was for.

One of the biggest hurdles was to try to remember how to get dressed. Living in a hospital, I never thought about clothes. Mary would help me look in the closet and drawers. I'd study things. I really had no memory of where pieces of clothes fit together.

Ever watch a two-year-old baby try to put on underpants? There are only three holes in them. If you're smart, you can figure out that one is bigger than the others. But front and back? That's interesting.

A bra, however, makes little sense to a child. And with aphasia, I had no awareness of my back as a part of my body. I could spend half an hour trying to dress, especially since looking in the mirror was unreal.

"You get dressed in the bathroom, April, not in the living room or the playroom."

"*Why?* It's easier in the big room," I said.

"People like to be private."

What! *Private?* Oh, well! By the time I got dressed, I was so tired I felt like a nap.

"Sorry, April. Keep your clothes on. You're going to St. Joe's for physical therapy."

To sit in a moving car was a bit like going on a roller coaster. I'd see a house zooming past me before I registered in my mind whose house that was. Our baby, in the back, was sleeping quietly. I was talking like a hyperactive child. It was at least a month before I realized Mary was driving me at about twenty-five miles an hour!

At St. Joe's they'd put me in a wheelchair and bring me to the P.T. rooms. In one room I would sit on a chair and exercise on the pulleys. Dr. Casey had me shake hands as hard as I could. I almost broke his hand. Strength I had, but no idea of how to handle it. The muscles of the back, the arm, and the fingers needed to be strengthened and to be moved with my mind.

The workers were more than competent. They sang with us, they laughed with us, and they helped us talk out some of our anger.

In another room I would be placed on a restorator, a contraption on which my knees and toes were moved as on a bicycle while I sat on a chair. Next to it, I would work at walking up and down two steps.

In between exercises I would sit in my wheelchair and rest. Occasionally I would be left somewhere apart from the P.T. team. Then I would grow very shy. I knew my first name. But if someone called for Mrs. Armstrong, I couldn't respond. I didn't know the surname. And if I was overtired, I would begin to believe that I would never communicate again.

Then, one day, feeling sorry for myself and crying, I suddenly saw an old friend, Frank Apicella, who entered in a wheelchair with his wife.

I cried: *What happened to you?*

He answered: *I had a stroke.*

His wife smiled sweetly. "Hello!"

Frank said: *You remember Mary?*

I said to Frank: *How could she be Mary? She is Mary.* I pointed to how petite Mary Apicella was. *But my Mary is thin and tall. She'll be right back here soon.*

Mary Apicella was talking to me, but I was not on her wavelength. I was excited.

I said to Frank: *You and I are talking the same language. Do you know Babel?*

*I don't know a Babel word,* said Frank. *But we sure can communicate.*

For the next five minutes he filled me in on the World Series, and Nixon. I was fascinated. He was several months ahead of me in aphasia. He could focus in on television, so he was cuing me in.

Then Mary Ball came in.

I said: *Frank, how can there be two Marys?*

Frank chuckled. *You'll learn. 'Member the Mothers' Circle? Mary and Mary Ball and Mary Walsh! I guess they sound the same.*

By that time Mary B. and Mary A. were listening and wondering.

"I don't understand what they're saying," said Mary A.

"They really have a different language," said Mary B.

"They really don't," said a volunteer.

"Oh, you think so? They mean it!" said Mary B.

"Babel," I said. "God knows that!"

Returning from physical therapy that day, I had lain down, wondering if all people with aphasia used the same language. Then, as clearly as before, I felt the Lord talking to me.

"You wanted to know about Babel?" said Jesus.

"Yes," I said.

"Simple people understand the language," said Jesus.

"Is it because we were put in a barrier, Lord?"

"No," said Jesus. "Words aren't necessary. *The Word is.*"

"I don't understand You," I said.

"In the beginning was the Word, and the Word was God," Jesus said, reminding me of the New Testament.

"You are the Word, Lord," I said.

"Then you understand, for you are simple. So many people know so many words, but they have forgotten listening, feeling, touching, hearing," said Jesus.

"I can't smell anything. And I cannot taste, Lord."

"You have enough to think about now," He said.

"Are there only the sick that know Babel, Lord?"

"No. Only those who are opened to be God's children. Some are great with words, and some are not. Some are dumb, or blind, or deaf. Some are physically healthy and some are not. But you can tell who are opened. Bow when you see them, and laugh with joy. They are My children," He said.

Right then I thought to myself that it was easier just communicating with aphasics. It would be easier, and I wouldn't have to learn how to read and write and talk English. But I didn't want to say that to the Lord.

"Don't be silly," said Jesus reprovingly.

I certainly couldn't get bored. I was, for example, trying to figure out how to eat with a fork, knife, and spoon, and also learned those words. After five years, knife and fork are still a little different for me, especially if I'm tired or busy. The hand and the right side of my body are such that if I don't concentrate I can eat with an upside-down knife carrying mashed potatoes to my mouth.

Mary kindly used to insist that I ask for things by name up till noon. Afternoons I could just point. And still Mary kept on talking to me about everything in the world, just as Paul and Martin did, mentioning simple words and big words. Martin would show me our books, our music boxes, our collections of memorabilia. Paul would tell me about rock-and-roll and games and school problems. Some I really remembered, and some I pretended to remember and obviously couldn't understand at all.

Obscured from me was the idea of male and female, father-mother, girl-boy. I did know there was a difference. But there was a short circuit in my brain; perhaps there was a cut made in operating on my brain? Who knows! But for three years I could not answer correctly whether the question was about a man or a woman. In my mind I knew who each person was. But to say it or write it, I was only 50 per cent correct. Add to that the pronouns "he" and "she," and my poor family and friends were frustrated. I could start out by saying *he* did something and then say *she* did something. To me, *he* and *she* were interchangeable. Then Martin or Mary would give up.

I was determined to learn the names of our family as quickly as possible. That would be easier than trying to say pronouns. So I would spend ten minutes at a time trying to spell their first names, and say them. But I was also interested in learning the difference between the ceiling and the floor, the window and the wall.

At least, resting on the bed, I knew where I was. My body was on terra firma. The right side of my body was cold, but it wouldn't fall or float away in bed. And lying down, I would close my eyes. It seemed to me that high over my head was my living computer, too far for me to reach it, but quite near enough for me to watch it. I knew myself, and I knew that the computer was still intact and growing. I believed that everything I had known was still complete. As I imagined it, I felt myself an astronaut returning from the most distant stars. I visualized myself as having been put into a compression chamber. The compression chamber was the time without language, and now I would have to relearn the language, to live again in the old world.

How do you grasp an idea, and bring it down from the stars to the conscious level in the brain? Lying down, I reached the computer, and grabbed one. *Charades!* Wordless, one can operate, and act out one's responses to another.

I went to the study, where Martin was paying some bills. I asked "Lady" what bills were for. He told me. I could not read or write, but as I looked at them I darn' well understood. Martin was naming them. I saw one and understood that one bill should not be mailed with money to an insurance company.

I stood, and got dizzy. I went back to bed. Charades was the way. I thought about it, and went back to the study. I picked up the bill, shook my head, put it down again, and tried acting. I motioned my left hand with three fingers. Then I tried to motion:

"Mmm hmm! Mmm hmm! Mmm hmm!"

"What are you doing? You want me to put a stamp on it? O.K."

I shook my head. Then I nodded, asking by motion to think of things.

"You sound silly. Oh—are you trying to play charades?"

"Yes!"

"But not insurance?"

"Yes!"

It took three nights before I could think of "waves." I did not know that "waiver" and "waves" would be different. But "water," "big water," meant to me not to put the stamp in the mail. Martin had mailed it, but I still wanted him to understand. As a teacher, I had bought an insurance policy for my retirement. Part of it meant that if I got sick I would not have to pay for my insurance premium.

Of course, Martin would have eventually realized this, and my good insurance agent would have told him about it. But I was gloriously proud of myself. I knew that for sure the aphasics could act things out, and so translate.

And that night, as I said my prayer, I said: "Thank you, Mary." And I meant Holy Mary, not Mary B. or Mary A. She was helping me to remember.

Meanwhile, on no-P.T. days, Pat Benzmiller had come to my house to play games with me. Checkers, I'd never really understood, even before I was sick. Chinese checkers, I liked. Candyland, a game for three-year-olds, was too difficult for me. I could and did play Go Fish. But, after half an hour, frustration took over.

I liked bridge, but I couldn't remember the suits or the numbers. I loved chess, but while I could remember how to use the knights, I had no memory of what pawns were for. Frustration!

I tried drawing a face. Psychiatrists would find it interesting. Like a three-year-old, I forgot about filling in the eyes.

I tried to write the Our Father. My mind remembered. By rote I could say most of it. But to write it out? The first word made no sense.

The sound was like "Are."

Mary B. wrote me the word "Our."

By rote the word was the same.

I gave up.

"Dear Lord, I am a prisoner clanging in the prison gate. God damn it, why?" I said.

Silence.

"Mary, help me. Hail, Mary, full of grace. . . ."

"Be still," said great Mary. "Don't fight it so hard. Accept it. It will be opened."

This had not happened before. I was scared, so I was still. Accept . . . *what?* What's going on?

"If you keep knocking at the door too hard, the door could suddenly be opened and you'd fall flat on the floor," she said, smiling. "Do you remember patience? You have a lot to learn."

"Mary, I always used to say that prayer from St. Louis de Montfort: Mary, speak in me and through me."

She was waiting.

"How can I say that if you are here? Or is it that you can help me when I learn patience? But what do I do with my worries? Am I crazy?"

"No."

"I wish I could have a good priest to talk with me. How do I

know if I'm seeing Jesus—and you—in a dream or real? I still
see—"

"The Three-in-One."

"The Trinity. Will it disappear?"

"You are so scared, dear. Be open and you will know," said
Mary. "You'll know what's true."

Who wants to come and talk to the disabled? In a way, they
mourn for the "living dead." Friends feel they should do something. But mourning is too difficult for many humans, too basic
beyond words. Yet, mourning is not very different from loving.
What is a wail? What is a deep, exultant laughter? What is silence? Basic aliveness. Opposites always exist when you are really alive.

But so few people remember how to feel anything. They
seem to be in a hurry, "on the way" and "by the way," traveling with no feet on the ground. These people are afraid of
things that are too happy to believe: birth, the winning streak,
growth. Is it jealousy, or personal sadness, that sends them
away? And the same people are afraid of things that are too
awful to believe: death, the destruction of an earthquake, the
sick and the handicapped at their lowest ebb.

Without warning to me, a good priest did come to talk with
me. I had not seen him for several years, when he moved to his
own Byzantine monastery in Ohio. With joy I remembered the
day of his ordination—Father George Applegate.

"I had to come back to the East for business, and on the
way I wanted to visit you. May I celebrate Mass here for your
recovery?"

Alleluia!

After Mass he sat in the playroom for four hours in almost silence, while I talked and talked and talked, and rested, and talked some more.

Could he understand what I was saying? Word-wise it was gibberish. My words were disjointed, and the more I wanted to tell him something the more stupidly would I talk. For me it was release. My joy, my confusion, my fears, calmed me. Instead of shaking the bars of my mind, I felt safe. I grew quieter and quieter.

I asked him questions. He said almost nothing. Bless him! As he sat for those hours, he accepted my glory and my loneliness, my frustration and my close friendship with the Lord. He accepted and joined them to his own. This is talking without words, when you do not know rationally what to say.

Father George knows what love is: the bread and drink of God. I have not seen him since then. But he gave me comfort and I pray for him often.

During those first few months, others came to bring me something, smile at me, and talk over me and around me to Mary B. and the family.

"Don't ask me," said Mary B. "Ask April if she's feeling better. Not me."

Friends swallowed nervously. How do you talk to somebody who has aphasia? Half of what I said made no sense. They did not want to discuss my embarrassment.

What I wanted to say was, Look, I'm still me.

But I'd get nervous and come out with "euphemisms." And friends left, being sure I had lost all my marbles.

Some came to talk to me about "poor April." Unreal! What they were really communicating to me was their own love of being sorry for themselves. They talked about their operations, and their worst times. They never found out how I felt about anything.

But with a real friend, Helen Mayglothling, I could understand the trauma of visiting someone you love. She had seen me in the hospital. She had called Martin regularly. And finally she came. Normally she would come into my house through the garage. Instead she went to the front door and rang the bell.

When she entered, she was talking a blue streak. Then, suddenly, she had nothing else to say. Mary B. went to get her some coffee.

"Hi, friend, it's me," I said, having learned some decent words.

"Say it again?" said Helen.

"Hi, friend." That was almost the end of my vocabulary. "Ceiling, floor, coffee."

Helen began to cry happily. Helen was not only an old, close friend but a speech teacher in the public school. "April, can I correct your mistakes as time goes on? Or should I just be polite and pretend not to hear them? I've been wondering about that for days."

"I me," I said.

"You mean: 'I'm me.'"

So we were hugging and crying and saying few words. And then, by coffeetime, we could be relaxed and normal. Helen had been a talker for twenty years, and she was again, and I loved it. There is no fear in being real.

That evening, I tried without words to formulate the fear of visiting the sick. Then, suddenly, my memory pictured a time when I visited a friend, Anna McDonnell, who was then suffering from senility. In a convalescent home, she remembered me, but her actions and words were wandering back in time. Five minutes later she would even forget that I had come. Ten minutes later, she was telling me what her brother was doing. Her brother, the bishop, was, of course, dead. I was scared, and polite. But I never came back to visit her. I thought of her often, and prayed for her.

But then I had believed there was no reason why I should come and sit with her.

Oh, God! I could not get angry at anyone for not visiting me. Tit for tat. I promised myself that from then on I would visit those incarcerated in Babel. I would talk. I would touch. I would be still, and accept the unsaid Word. Unafraid.

I wept for Anna McDonnell, who died before I could learn that lesson.

My memory of her helped me in another way. I began to wonder why I was crying so much. Doctors had said that most aphasics overact in their emotions. Could it be instead that we are just *re*acting to awareness, as all people should do? So-called normal people have learned to be "cool," to swallow awareness. But we are given a second chance. With laughter, we cry. With joy, we cry. With sadness, we cry. Childlike, we are never disinterested. We feel life.

If I had to choose between being disinterested and cool, and overreacting, I'd swear for full aliveness!

At P.T. at St. Joe's, the therapist was gradually adding more weights on my feet as I worked on the restorator. I would have sworn those weights were about fifty pounds. Actually, they were only three pounds. Numbers meant nothing to my brain. All I knew was that the exercises were a bit painful and a real bore.

So I'd start trying to think of almost anything else. Mary Ball had taught me part of the alphabet.

"A B C D E F G!" I sang, flat and loud.

Frank Apicella was exercising near by.

"A B C D E F!" I sang again.

"Find another song," said Frank. "For God's sake, find another song."

"1 2 3 4 5!"

"Don't you want to talk?" asked Frank. "How about football?"

"I don't know how to play football—or watch it," I said.

"Then, maybe it's time for you to do something else!" said Frank.

And of course, at P.T., it was always time to do something else. It was time for me to take off the weights and work on walking up and down the stairs. The game was to walk up two steps with only one hand touching the rail, cross the small landing, and go down the other side.

The first time I did it, I nearly fell. I was showing off, and I had not noticed that the steps on one side were different from the steps on the other side.

Terrified, I wondered why they made them with different sizes. Why the hell do you do that to patients?

The therapist explained. "So you will learn to watch your steps. You have to learn to judge distance."

I swallowed my retort. Words couldn't help. Like a child, the aphasic could not visualize distance. It had to be felt, physically telling the body where things belong. To co-ordinate walking, stepping, standing, and seeing is a big job.

What I wanted to do was to get out of P.T. and into speech with the pathologist. To me it was more important to learn to read than play around with P.T. I noticed that Ben Cariri and other speech teachers came to meet their patients in the hospital. Why didn't that happen for me?

Dr. Casey explained. "April, I won't let you go to school until you have learned how to get your muscles working. There's no easy way to skip regrowing. It affects your eyes, your body, your brain, and your mind. Everything."

Oh, euphemism!

"How about some more pulleys next time? And now let's have you walk all over these rooms without holding on?"

Dr. Casey understood Babel. Casey was a real doctor, who consoled a patient by leading him into really higher achievements. That's a difficult game. Casey spoke to each patient as a friend. In some unusual way, he gave the patient a sense of honor. "I am a good doctor, and you know it. So in this part, I am trying to help you. But you are a good person, and I know it. So you must also try to help me. And you can tell me, and share it with me."

Casey was teaching me, physically and emotionally. Physically I kept on with P.T. Emotionally I was trying to learn patience and master each new day's growth. The yoke is easy and light when you don't fight against it.

The day did come when I could go to school. Martin drove me to the entrance of Ben Cariri's office, and I walked my way in proudly. Martin had gone to park the car. I sat down on the nearest chair I could see. Slowly I focused on the chair, and the office. Then, from another room, I heard a man and a child coming toward me.

I instantly knew I should not be sitting in this office. Part of deep aphasia is the slowness of the brain. Darkness and confusion envelop the unknown. I wanted to run away, but I couldn't.

"April, I'm Ben Cariri. Can I help you move to a more comfortable chair in the waiting room?"

"Mmm hmm," I said. I felt his hand, and fear fell apart as he led me to the waiting room I had not even noticed. But as Martin came in I said: "Lady, I love Ben. Hooray!"

Speech pathologists and speech teachers need a good sound as they speak. And they need empathy for their patients. Just like doctors, they may be good at their craft, and doing their duty, but to win the whole trust of the patient they also need a person-to-person awareness. To be competent without love is almost useless. Yet they also have to be cool, to be firm.

Until my illness, I had thought only of children's speech problems, reading, and writing. My friend Helen worked largely with dyslexics, stutterers, and autistic children. She was deeply involved in each student.

"It's a sticky line," Helen had said to me once. "You can't be a mother, worrying about each child. But you can't close your memory of a child when a half-hour appointment is over. I can't go home talking to my Bud constantly, especially since confidentiality is important to each family. It is like being a lawyer or a priest. But your mind mulls on the child even while you're asleep. And next day, when you teach him again, you get to understand what ESP is for. And there is a bridge growing from the teacher to the child."

I was lucky to have fine speech teachers. I have watched others working and wanted to cry out, "Drop the façade, and look in the heart of the patient! You can see her faults. Can you see her dignity frozen inside her? Can you pray, in your own way, to feel how you'd feel in her shoes?"

If language controls your ability to communicate, pick the best speech teacher for yourself. If I had my way I'd pay speech teachers as high as surgeons. (Of course, I believe all teachers should be paid as high as physicians.) Language is the opening to human life. And aphasics sense that language is not rote, and is not something to be simply taught, but a fullness of soul.

How did you learn English? By growing in the roots and soul of a family. You learned basic English before you ever got to school with a teacher. How did you *lose* English in a stroke? By being unrooted. Your speech teacher is partly involved in helping you through school. But a good speech teacher is also trying to bridge your soul back into normal life. The use of your religion has nothing to do with it. But the use of all senses —mind, soul, and body—must work together.

I put my trust first in Ben Cariri.

"What do you want to do?" said Ben.

"To read. To write."

"And 'rithmetic," said Ben.

I shook my head.

"You have to, April. You had a pyramid of language. And the pyramid fell down. To rebuild it, you must take one step at a time. To talk, to read, to write. You must also learn numbers, and multiplication, and division. Or the whole pyramid falls down again."

I was darn' contrary. I was never good at math. I liked algebra, and never really understood geometry.

"One, two, three, four, five, six—is that enough?" For years, the seven's upset me.

"No," said Ben. "Sorry about that. If you want to buy something, you'll need money. Right? If you want to pay, you must learn how much to get back."

He took the change from his pocket and put it on the table.

Oh, God! I hadn't thought about money. There was lots of change. More than five. Tears came from my eyes. Slowly I was learning how much I didn't know. How the hell could anyone start over? I halfway had believed that I could study a bit and start reading normally. And now?

"April, do you remember what it was like looking at the library catalogues? You remember looking up a card in the catalogue?"

"Yes." My mind flashed that message.

"Aphasia means somebody dropped all the cards on the floor."

"Yah!" You mean really? "Yuk!"

"Together, you and I will pick them up and put them back in the trays."

"One by one?" I started to cry again.

"Sometimes they come in bunches. And sometimes one by one. Now—we'll talk more about it another day. But for now I want to start helping you. And you've got to learn first to know where you're at."

I said, "Ceiling. Floor. Window. Wall."

"Show me the wall?"

I had no idea, really. I had been learning the words by rote. And being a smart kid, I watched when Mary B. or Martin would say the word. They always looked toward the sound. So I answered.

Ben laughed. "No wonder you're smart. But my job is to trick you a bit, until the sound gets into your mind. Here is a wall. Show me another one."

I wondered: How could there be another wall?

"Touch it. Feel it. This is a wall."

I touched a wall with a window.

"There is a wall. Up to here is a wall. In it is a window."

"Why?" I was beginning to use *Why* constantly, like a child. As a mother I sometimes thought I was being teased. Now I understood. The child is baffled with language, and keeps hoping to understand.

"*Why?* Why did a wall come together with another wall?"

And like a child, an aphasic could quickly lose interest.

Ben was beginning to teach me the parts of the body. The leg, the knee, the foot. The back, the chest, abdomen. The shoulder, the arm, the hand.

"The shoulder," said Ben.

"The soldier," I said.

By the third time, it suddenly dawned on me. When I was a child I was having trouble learning the word *shoulder*. In my memory, I saw the place where I lived in New York City on the West Side. I lived in a brownstone house. My Mummy knew my problem with *shoulder*.

"Ben—I 'member Mummy an' shol'er."

"Hold on to it," said Ben. "If your memory is returning, you may find it easier looking for words. But some words have to be learned by rote. It's like learning a new language without any roots and no dictionary."

I was to take a list of body words and have Mary B. quiz me five times a day. I went home with trust and—time for a nap— almost exhausted. Learning language is the most difficult exercise in the world, taxing on the brain.

With physical therapy you know what the goal is. It can be measured. You walk from here to there. You jump, or try to. You move your body and either you make it or you don't. In language, you are reliving your memory. You are singing half-remembered songs. You are reeling, staggering with ideas without moving.

And if, as an aphasic, your eyes cause problems, you are in a mass of visual confusion. In me the eye itself was all right. But the nerves in the middle of the head were disturbed. I saw everything as two-dimensional, flat, as on a postcard. In addition, I saw people as if they were painted by Picasso, with one eye huge and one sideways. And part of each eye had a void. Doctors have their own medical jargon. But it was easier to explain it by saying that where there is a void in the eye, there is a bit of nothing. And the brain does not like voids. Some deaf people have a void in sounds, and their brain often turns on music or words that do not exist. Blind people visualize. I closed my eyes without visualizing. Two parts of my mind continued visualizing: a place in the upper right corner of my eyes, where I could never fully see the picture. And if I opened my eyes I saw three fifths of what was really there, one fifth filled with gigantic Picasso images of what was real, and one fifth filled with a void of any visualized idea that was running in my brain.

If, for example, I had been looking at the Van Gogh picture in Ben's office and then looked at him or at the table, on the right side of my eye I still saw a part of that picture. To try to read, or write, or move was a damned nuisance.

Aphasics need much rest after working on words in speech therapy. But they have one joy many people have forgotten: the glory of awareness without words.

The world is wondrous. And aphasics are forced to see the beauty. The sun, the rain, the first star; the look of a bird, and a rat, and a spider—the sounds of life overwhelmed me. I would sit in a chair and watch a tree, day after day, until I began to understand the tree and the little rat that lived under a rock, and Poltergeist and I and Mary Ball and Martin and Paul are in union with life. The past, the present, and the future melt in God.

"Do you see it!" I wanted to say. "Jump in it to silence."

But how could anyone say: Jump into silence? I did not know how to explain it to others. In aphasia, one is meditating constantly. But without words, how could I translate it for others?

I knew I needed help. I wanted to get in touch with a well-known psychiatrist, Dr. Jean Houston, who would understand my problem. I played charades with Martin, and in a few days we had focused on her name and address. Martin called her for me. Dr. Houston sent a friend to help me, a man who was traveling toward New York, and he would be interested in meditating during the convalescing of aphasia.

"Pepper?"

"His name is Peper," said Martin.

Pepper and salt has to do with eating, and I was learning

that word at school. How could there be a man called Peper? I kept hoping I would try to hear the name Peper correctly, while Martin kept telling me the sound was the same. It was as horrible to me as saying Mary and Mary and Mary, and not knowing why. My brain was zipping around in my brain. Thank God! Dr. Peper came and knew a lot about aphasia. He held my hand, and told me to relax.

"Jean Houston said you used to meditate. Let's see how much you remember. Get yourself comfortable. Really comfortable. Don't wear anything too tight. Don't feel cramped. Lie down on the bed."

I nodded.

"Now take a few deep breaths."

My eyes grew frightened.

"You can't remember the word 'breath'? That's all right. You will remember," said Dr. Peper.

"No."

"Yes, you do. You're scared because you are trying to learn words. Your body has been hurt, so it can't remember correctly. So watch me. I'll act out a deep breath. Were you a singer at a church? Ah! Fill yourself with air, hold it, and let it go until all the old air gets out."

I smiled.

"Then again, April. I want you to relax so much that you can't tell the difference between you and the bed. Then, for two minutes I want you to let go and do nothing."

Two minutes to relax? Typical. After an instant I kept waiting for the two minutes to appear. But then I remembered. Gently my mind remembered, slowed myself, to a deeper level.

Then, quietly, Dr. Peper asked me to remember a special place I had in my inner peace. For me, it was a place next to the ocean. To reach it, I would picture myself walking up to the dunes, till finally I felt the breath of the sea. There I could visualize the sand, the water, the ocean, and the heavens. There I could visualize myself moving easily, singing where no one could hear me, crying a welcome to the world.

Quietly, Dr. Peper was asking me to remember the way of reaching a more comfortable level in the brain.

"Did you always stand at the seashore?"

"No." I remembered that to meditate well you were free of worries, money, or climate. I would sit on the sand and listen to the sounds of the sea. I was always warm. And when it was necessary I could visualize a shelter, a silent jetty, with a good chair.

"Two minutes, April, to make your deepest level happy in your place. It is a place where you can keep things together. It's a place where you can see everything. Yes? Two minutes, till you feel totally ready to reach an even lower level."

I no longer visualized it. I would say I was in it.

Slowly Dr. Peper called to me. "Now, you stand apart and look at your body. Feel it. Touch it in your mind. The blood is running through it. The arteries are strong and clear. The muscles are relaxed. See your fingers? See your toes? Visualize them, and accept them. This is you. Not bad. Not good. Just you."

Eyes closed. I yawned.

"Start up in your head, and slowly feel yourself. Whether you have words or not, it doesn't matter. But you know your body. Visualize it, all the way to your toes. For two minutes."

I was still busy feeling my knee when the time passed.

"Now, remember, there is no rush. As days pass you will get the sense of time. But move on now to the whole feeling of your body. Tell yourself of the great work that is being done to help you. Visualize Dr. Ray, who operated on your body, and healed it with strong plastic to keep your brain busy. Dr.

Nagle, who takes care of your medicines. Dr. Casey and the therapist. Ben healing you with words and speech. Believe in them, and tell yourself how much healing is being done."

Two minutes, and he continued. "Now turn and feel the changes going on in your body itself. Visualize your legs and arms growing stronger, making connections in your body, so you will be moving better. Visualize your brain taking the library cards picked up and neatly organized. Visualize your eyes, especially your right eye, healing, to make it easier to read. Two minutes."

I visualized, knowing then that only by deep relaxation could I bear to believe.

"Now. It is time to go to another level. To the mind of God. To thank Him. To praise Him. To talk to Him."

Two minutes later, Dr. Peper said: "And now—be nothing. For a few minutes be totally silent. Then open your eyes. You will feel very alive."

Which, of course, was true. I was more refreshed than I had been for weeks.

I tried to explain to Dr. Peper what had been happening to my brain.

"Don't worry about words. Just say it. And I'll translate it back to be sure of what you're saying."

I thought of my brain as having four levels: Alpha, Beta, Theta, and Delta. I thought of Beta as the lowest level of the brain, the level where you handle routine jobs, like answering the phone or making a cake. To me, Delta was the level where you were asleep, with the unconscious level in charge, and the involuntary work of the body was busy mending you.

Dr. Peper understood what I was saying, whether he agreed or not.

Now, I said, Alpha was the level I usually used to live on. It was a level of studying, hearing, and growing on an ESP level.

But with Theta I could move to the level of meditation. Only, I had forgotten where I was.

Dr. Peper renumerated. "If I accept your model, I will try to tell you where your problem is. In your mind, aphasia and the operation either numbed your brain or Beta was lost. You have to relearn it, by speech. And you know how to work at it.

"But Delta is not lost, just numbed. Your problem is to work on Delta much harder. You are busy, wanting to read and write. But the basic level is to know your body and to be proud of it. Don't be too busy growing up, the second time around."

The same thing—from Dr. Casey, from Ben Cariri. I groaned.

"Aphasics have to be childlike. And that's good."

I was silent. Then I said, "Will I make it?"

"If you want to."

I started to say: I've got to! And then my whole body and soul said instead, "I want to."

"In your brain, and in every man's head, are thousands of cells never used. They're there to be used. All you have to do is to get a connection from one idea to another. In meditating on Delta, and on Beta, use the extra cells. It'll take time, but you can do it."

A year ago I would have explained it in a more grown-up way. I would have talked about synapses, where the nerve impulses to the brain are passed on from one neuron to another. But "cells" were easier for me to visualize. Whether we agree about Alpha-Beta meditation or not, we all agree that there are ways of relearning language skills. It's like having a telephone wire. With aphasia, your line is disconnected. Your wire is burnt out. But there is room for other lines into your room. All you have to do is believe that eventually it will be spliced.

After five years, I have some pieces spliced together. But I'm not through.

And I still thank Dr. Peper for putting me back on the right track. There are many ways of meditating, of course. But I believe that all aphasics are forced to reach the lower levels of their brain. What I would call "Beta" is the most difficult job for them, to relearn language skills. But they need assurance to accept and use the other levels of the mind, from the unconscious level to the meditation level to the ESP level. It's like receiving a great gift—and not knowing it is there.

I would go to speech twice a week with Ben, and I would bring my homework like a good kid. I was printing the first names of myself and family and friends, and God. I was printing the street where I lived, but the phone number was very difficult.

Then Ben would use flash cards for me to name out loud.

"Coat," he would say.

"Coat." Part of me was wondering whether I could remember French. The word "coat" as Ben said it did not sound to me like *coat*. The word *coat* looked disoriented.

He showed me a *cup*. Inside myself I wanted to say *"clef."* No word came out. I tried *cup*. No sign. I tried Latin and German.

*"Ich weis' nich'."*

Ben looked interested. "Sing it. Songs return to the brain from your earliest childhood. But they will not help you in learning words. It's a different part in the brain."

I sang a song of Schiller, with words missing.

"Good. Now try to think about 'cup.'"

No real answer.

"Cup," said Ben. "Want a cup of coffee with me?"

"Cup . . . o' . . . coffee."

We went to another room as he made instant coffee. He found that I talked better when I felt I was on a break, relaxing. Speech teachers are sleuths, learning to guess what words are left out when aphasics talk. The so-called break for coffee was Ben's way of calming my mind, and guessing what daily words I most wanted to use.

"I want to buy things," I said. "And I will, damn it."

"A store? Clothes?"

"No."

Ben mentioned many. He said something and I pondered. The sound had no real ring to me. With the cup of coffee in my hand, I walked into the waiting room and looked at the magazines. *Sports Illustrated, Psychology Today, Glamour.* I felt sad.

"That's my fault," said Ben. "I haven't brought in more magazines, and some people took a lot of them away."

Searching, I found a page that looked like a big map. I showed it to Ben.

"Map?" he said. "You want a map?"

"Map. Big."

"You want to buy one?"

I laughed. I mimicked writing the word on a piece of paper.

"I'll write it down. But I bet you don't just want a map. You want that to do something else?"

I nodded.

"If I know you, you will. When you come here next week, you'll tell me what you really want to buy. And now, before you leave this time, let's work on the days of the week, and the months of the year, and the ABC's."

When Mary B. picked me up, Ben gave her a piece of paper.

"Map," I said. "Buy something."

"Map? Ben, I've brought her to stores, and what she wants is not in any stores here in Stamford. But why a map?"

"April," said Ben. "You want a map to get to know something else? Then, say it out loud, even if it sounds wrong."

"K'apo'kin."

No recognition by Mary or Ben.

"O.K. We'll get a big map. And she'll play charades. And she'll finally reach us."

In New York, Martin bought me a beautiful large world map and hung it in the playroom. I pointed out Russia.

"You really don't want all Russia. Twenty questions?"

I tried looking at Russian cities, looking for K, hoping it would work. My eyes were terribly tired.

"You did a lot already. Don't work so hard. It's a long day. You'd better get to bed," he said.

"O.K. But—" I smiled radiantly. "Meditation. Before sleep."

"You said that word so clearly," said Martin.

I got into my pajamas. I knew I was so very tired that it would be stupid for me to try to brush my teeth. I'd put Crest on my left finger and hope for the best. Then in bed I turned on the tape recorder and let Dr. Peper tell me how to reach the lower levels of my brain.

Martin came in about twenty minutes later. He thought I was asleep and turned off the tape. I opened my eyes.

"Thanks, Martin."

He looked about ready to cry.

I sat up in bed. "Martin! No more 'Lady'! I said: Martin!"

Even Poltergeist barked.

With twenty questions and charades, I had, by the next night, told them it was about a well-known name in this generation. It was not the czar. It was not a Communist. It sounded like "K."

Then, since I couldn't remember the alphabet, I was stymied. I started on a new tack. Ben had been teaching me to write the word *Stamford*. So I tried to write that down. Mary Ball corrected it after I wrote it.

"Say *Stamford*."

"O.K. *Stamford*. But No!"

"Nearby? Darien? New Canaan?" asked Mary.

Words didn't stick in my brain. I grabbed her and pointed toward the north.

"Let's go!" said Mary. It was late in the day, but we and the baby got in the car. "Show me."

It was New Canaan I wanted, and Mary insisted that I learn how to say that word. And I pointed the way until we ended up at one of the prettiest gift shops in the world.

"Kropotkin? No wonder you couldn't spell it!"

"Kropotkin!"

Back in the spring of that year I had found that gift shop in a quaint old house. I had been struck with the personal kindness of the owner and the workers. Florence Alden had an almost forgotten art of selling. Drop in, and they offer you a cup of coffee or tea while you browse. There were gifts from fifty cents up, with salespeople who were interested in helping you, not by price but by putting themselves in your shoes.

I found Florence. She could not remember me, but she realized I was not well. She found me a chair and gave me some coffee.

"I don't talk well," I said.

She looked at Mary and the baby. "April doesn't need help from me. If she got us here, she'll manage it. The place is beautiful, so I'll look around."

Suddenly I remembered my head. With a strange crew cut, and the left side of the head still almost bald, any woman would think I was a bit odd. I wondered if it would upset others shopping in the store. But kindness shone through Florence.

"Is there anything special you want? A present?"

I nodded. As quickly as I could, I sang the song without the words.

"Happy birthday! You need a happy birthday present. For a child?"

"No. Two. A big and a big." I acted out a tall one and a taller one.

Quickly she narrowed it down. The loss of words on male and female, son and father caused confusion, but she was good as a charade person, too.

"One for your son. One for your husband." I was tired, and drank my coffee. In a few minutes she put before me nine different, unique, and handsome presents for me to pick from. I burst out crying with happiness, selecting one for each. But as she began wrapping them with a red and white mushroom on the bow, I suddenly got worried.

"Mary?"

"I know," said Mary. "I didn't know why you wanted to go here, and I'm short on cash. But—"

Ben had said I would have to learn what money was. But Florence looked at me.

"We'll charge it for you. I do remember you. And just because you have problems, don't be scared. If you ever need help here, call me up." She chuckled. "We do at times make an evening appointment for people who are unwell."

How many special stores would take care of such problems? For aphasia, at least, the gift of quietness and understanding is rare. The amount of money I've spent at Kropotkin's was hardly worth the store's time. But the people working there were in a one-to-one awareness of life.

On the way home, I hugged the birthday presents in my left hand. It was late, and we were hurrying home and not just for dinner. With aphasia, darkness is riding in a Kafka nightmare.

It is not just the problem of bright lights passing a car. Without good vision the brain panics.

Mary turned on the inside light in the car, and quietly tried to turn me away from fear. "Don't forget to make notes in your mind about Kropotkin's. Imagine getting a map to think of Russia? It's only four minutes till you'll be home."

"Car's cold. I won't cry."

"As a reporter, April, make a note. And since you can't write, you'll have to remember. And that will keep you busy as we drive home in the cold dark."

She brought me home and suggested that I have a snooze till Martin came home. I didn't want to sleep. I held on to my presents and sat in the dark. Then I lit a cigarette, to make unwritten notes.

By God, it was true. In the dark the red light of the cigarette danced. I knew the cigarette was in my left hand. I turned that hand farther to the left. My brain saw the cigarette move leaving a slow trace of the orange-red line. Why? A lazy eye? So many questions! I turned on the light. Now I didn't have a lazy eye?

By then I was getting comfortably warm. Why did I get so terribly cold in the car? Is it just because it was getting toward winter? I remembered. The right side of my body was always cold. Was it circulation?

"What-cha doing?" said Martin.

I gave him his present.

"I already had my birthday!" he said happily.

I pointed to the map, and sang the song. By mime, I told him and my son, Mike, it wasn't a real birthday till I could buy them presents all by myself.

Christmas brought the family together. In many ways I was excited and happy. But in many ways, like other aphasics, I could hardly stand it. There was too much of everything.

Noise is a real pain in the head. Normal people cannot really understand it. For two months our house had been quiet. But if two people talked at the same time, I would get nervous. If they also talked while the stereo was on, I felt a shaking, and moved quickly to another room.

By this time Martin of course had studied quite a bit on aphasia, but it was clear that doctors and their pamphlets said little of normal problems with families.

Daughter Cathy came before Christmas, bringing me the thrill of finally seeing her child, Ginny King. I looked and wondered, but I did not really caress her or cuddle her.

Mary Ball watched me. "You haven't really touched the foster-home child either."

I wouldn't touch either one. I was polite, and afraid. God knows what psychological hang-up is there. It was not that I wanted to be the most important child around. My other grandchild, Jenny, was a year older than Ginny. And she could walk. But a lying-down child? Others cuddled them. But I was sure I could break them.

Besides . . . I really did not understand where babies came from, or how they operated.

When I saw Jenny and Ginny together, frustration intensified. Part of it was noise. Part of it was wondering about babies in general. And worst of all, the problem of names. I had a daughter, Cathy. I had a daughter-in-law, Kathy. And two grandchildren, Jenny and Ginny. C-K and G-J. My language skills were shot. To picture their names, to hear their names, drove me up the wall. I couldn't remember what a wall was, either. I loved them all and ended up crying.

Would the world never become stable?

Martin and Mary agreed that I should stay mostly in the playroom and relax in quietness. But no matter what I did, I made a mess.

I loved getting ready for Christmas. At Kropotkin's, I had

bought my gifts. I loved wrapping presents, and did a fairly good job. Then I began signing the cards, and showed them to Mary Ball.

Four presents, wrapped and signed.

"To April from Mary and Bud."

To me that made perfect sense. As I saw it, the first name was the giver and the second name was the receiver.

"*To* and *from* are different prepositions," said Mary.

"To too?"

Mary said, "Just put your own name on every present and we'll all understand. You're printing it *so* well!"

"But I want it right!"

Daughter Clare, home for vacation, had been working with me on learning nursery rhymes. That was, after all, part of homework for my speech teacher.

"Wow! You wrapped your presents already. That's more than I've done." She looked at the cache of wrapped presents. "You've bought all those presents—"

I saw her face. She was afraid to look at me.

"Tell me. Again. Tell me."

"O.K., Mom. Did you buy those presents for you? No? Did you buy them for others? Yes? Then, change the names."

"Why? Me? You?" Despair. I sat in a corner and felt like dying. I was shaking.

Mary Ball and Clare brought me a bowl of ice cream.

"Ever get angry?" said Mary.

With tears streaming down my face I wanted to send the ice cream all over Mary's nose—except that I liked chocolate, so I held onto it.

"You want a good job? It's time to get rid of frustration."

After I ate the ice cream, she led me to the cabinets in the kitchen.

"Open them. Then close them with all the strength you've

got." She showed me, and she hit the cabinet so hard that the next cabinet opened.

"Go right around the cabinets, banging them hard!"

I did the first one halfheartedly. Nothing exciting. Then I tried it again, harder, harder. That made the one on the right open. I slammed it, and the next one opened.

What joy! Around and around I went, four times around the kitchen. My body was so full of frustration, the muscles so tense, that the release of anger was beautiful. By the fifth time around, I started to laugh.

By that time the whole family was watching. The foster-home baby and Cathy's baby were crying. The dogs were barking. But joy reigned.

The day after Christmas, I was able to say the names of my seven children and spell them.

Alleluia!

Bad words were gone, except Hell and God damn it. Good words, I was learning. I knew how to get dressed and I could take my own shower. I could *give* presents without worrying about prepositions.

I felt safe with beautiful people.

And in January I was to go to New York to see Dr. Ray, the neurosurgeon.

"I'm going with New York!" I said.

To? From? With? For? Who cared? "I am going out to the open world," I answered, and went to bed to meditate.

## CHAPTER FIVE

"I'm going to see my neurosurgeon. It's 1973! I've got an appointment to get a checkup with Dr. Bronson Ray." Those words struck me so deeply! Indeed, in that year, January, June, and December, there would be three different chords as the healing in the brain continued in aphasia.

The first time, I felt nervous-happy-disappointed all at the same time. Typical of aphasia after a few months, my inner being felt like putting my toe in the water, to find out whether I liked this world's reality. I had been told that Dr. Ray was famous. As I understood it, he had invented the procedure of opening the brain, cleaning the hemorrhage, and filling the space with hard plastic material. I had been told that he had saved my life.

Aphasics are truthful and simple, and therefore impolite. One reason I was anxious to meet him was to tell him something important: "For your next operation, don't shave the hair off on only one side of the head." But first things first.

On the drive into New York, I was cogitating my feelings. I had no memory of ever seeing Dr. Ray until I saw him during the operation. Obviously he had seen me, but as a reporter, I must say I did not see him until I sat on a ledge over the operating room looking down on the scene. I saw the group working on me and found it hard to see their faces, because they were looking down on me. I did, however, see the most important doctor in the group walking out. I was afraid. But then he returned.

Some weeks later, recuperating at home, I was still worried about his leaving the scene. Dr. Al Dunn explained to me that, in operations over eight hours, even doctors need to go to the bathroom. I chuckled. But Dr. Al was interested in knowing why I thought I could see him from up on the ledge.

I wanted to tell Dr. Ray about that, too. But, mostly, I wanted to see what he really looked like. The day after the operation, I had seen him, but the clearest way to report that is to say I saw him two different ways. My eyes were blurry. Visually, I saw Dr. Ray as of middle height, in his sixties, happy. He was saying that I would go to therapy and see him in about three months. On another level of the brain, I saw a picture of my obstetrician, Dr. Duke Damon, and had a clear understanding that it was not Damon but, rather, like him. Dr. Ray was kind, brilliant, and proud of his work. That picture is still sharp in my memory, because in the brain it was like watching two films spread one over the other: Damon at my legs during a delivery, and Ray standing next to my head. I wanted to explain that to Dr. Ray, the mysterious ways the brain uses to communicate.

Oh, so many things I wanted to say to him this January of 1973. But I could hardly talk correctly at all. He was good-looking, kind, and fantastic as a doctor. But how do you say thank you? With so many feelings, my mind went quite blank. Martin and Dr. Ray talked about my medicines, my physical therapy, my speech. At commands, I walked and turned like a robot.

Then Dr. Ray led me to a room and placed some objects on the table. "Can you name any of these?"

I studied them: a thimble, a penny, a quarter, a rubber band, a paper clip, a nut and bolt, a bobby pin. Tears welled in my eyes.

"Can you show me how to use something with this?"

I picked up the money and mimed it into my pocket.

"Good. Anything else?"

I was furious. I knew I never used a thimble, and could care less about nuts and bolts. I picked up a rubber band and stretched it, as if to use it as a sling. I wished to kill him with it. He watched very closely. "April, shake my hand." I knew that I had hurt Dr. Casey's hand. Dr. Ray accepted my hand. "You nearly broke my hand. Don't do that to a nice old man. You're young, you'll survive. But me?"

I felt better.

He led me to his office. "Two things you have to do every day. One is to read the newspaper." I started to feel sorry for myself. "Whether you can read it or not, look at it. Turn the pages. You must! Just co-ordinating, handling the papers, looking at the pictures, knowing you will be able to read."

"O.K."

"Do you know how to play bridge? Do you like it?"

I loved bridge. In college I had found it to be an addiction. Married and working, I seldom played, but I always read about it in the newspapers. Now, I thought, since I couldn't work I could finally play.

"Some of my patients find it great. And my great bridge expert, who still can't write well or talk well, is a real winning master. Puts together co-ordination, numbers, memory concentration—I order you to play."

There must be a reason. In all those five years, I still haven't played. I had not taught the family how to play before I got sick. And like most families with aphasics, there isn't time to learn a new game. Perhaps therapy groups could try it on recreation time.

Listening to Dr. Ray, I knew he was a beautiful man, and I wanted so much to tell him how I felt. "If you had to fix me," I said slowly, "thank you." It would take another two years before I could explain it to others. I said it again and again, and wrote it down when I got home.

The next day, we were having a coffee klatch. Mary Ball and Pat Benzmiller and I were on a break from doing my "homework" on naming the whole alphabet, and writing "Dan sat on a mat." I looked at these beautiful friends and felt safe.

"I've wanted to ask you something. Help me!"

"Sure, you know you have wonderful problems." They were smiling, stirring the coffee. But they knew then I was a bit nervous.

"I have seven children," I said. "But, please—where did they come from?" I looked at Mary and Pat and I saw that they were a bit hesitant. "I remember knowing about getting periods. I've been trying to remember where these two pieces go together. But I can't remember what my mother had said." Mary and Pat glanced at each other, looking a bit red, and burst out roaring with laughter. Then they turned away, as if running in different directions. Then they looked at me.

"Oh, April!" said Mary. "Hey, this is great. Do you remember teaching Marriage at SHU? You were teaching nurses at St. Vincent's, and an elective course at SHU? Oh, boy, April."

"No," I said.

"I remember," said Mary. "You used to say that you wished people with so many hang-ups could be taught correctly the first time. Do you remember how sad you felt for girls in college who were afraid they could become pregnant from a kiss?"

By then, Pat and Mary were talking to each other. "Remember when April said that four girls in her class thought babies came out from the navel?" Then it sank into their minds. I started to cry, quietly; I had a blank. So we talked for about an hour. I was fascinated with sex. Finally, I said, "Poor Martin! But why didn't he tell me?"

"Sex right after an operation? Even people with heart attacks have to wait for a while. He was probably told by the doctors to wait until you felt ready."

Now, writing in retrospect, I believe it necessary to mention this to all who know aphasics, because doctors and therapists do not begin to notice the nuances of the patient's sexual needs, so they fail to help the patient or the family. Sex is always one of the deepest levels of life.

And Babel exists everywhere.

A few days later, I was in St. Patrick's Cathedral, about ten rows from the main altar. Something kept making me wonder what was going on next to me. I was sitting in a left-side pew and I couldn't see clearly on my right side. I turned. At first I thought I saw a casket coming forward, as if funeral bearers were carrying something nearer to the altar. I thought I saw tall candles and a huge casket, but it wasn't. Just a man was there. Nothing else.

I sat back to meditate. Then I turned to the right again. Jesus was there. He was kneeling in the center aisle. Kneeling? I knelt. I had never thought of Him as kneeling after Resurrection.

"Pray with Me," He said. "Don't pray to Me. Pray with Me." Then He was silent. I looked at Him from His back. He was ahead of us, but He was on our side, not in the sanctuary. "I need you all!" said Jesus. "Oh, I need you."

I shuddered.

"Pray with Me to our Father! Our Father in heaven. We hallow your name. Your kingdom come! Your will, Father, be *done!*"

Silent, I could stop shaking. "I wish there could be a large statue of You," I said. "Not over the altar, not in a niche, but ahead of us, teaching us how to pray to Him. I'd like a sculptor to make it in every church. With that we could feel close and sure, as You teach us how to pray."

He looked back at me over His shoulder.

"I would kneel under Your elbow," I said.

"Climb up on My back," said Jesus.

"No," I said. "That would be rude."

He burst into laughing with me. "Poor child," He said. "I carry all children. You're not grown up. Get up on Me piggyback."

I held my head, as if exploding. This is unreal. That's not what God is?

"I am nestling all people, as though brooding over My chickens. Why don't you believe it? Why don't others believe Me? Father—why?" asked Jesus.

"I'm too scared, Lord," I said. "Even as a little child I was scared with my father. I might fall."

"Even with Me? Break through being polite. You don't believe God all the way. Hold tight and walk with Me."

I still felt uneasy. I wanted so much to talk to a special priest. Even my children could figure out who I wanted to talk to when I said, "The man who put his yellow cap on his beard when he swam in our pool at the party." Father George Maloney, s.j. Martin wrote him at Fordham.

"He's awful busy," said Martin kindly. "He's always giving retreats and giving talks all over the country."

The problem of confession for the sick is different, especially for aphasics. Babel—the lack of communication—rests in the patient who hopes one understands. There is a real cry of fear for those who believe in One God, the Three-in-One, and are prisoned, afraid of the worst sin of all, blasphemy against the Spirit.

The telephone rang. It was my close friend who is a cloistered Dominican nun. I, who still had a real problem talking over the phone, became excited when Mary Ball told me the call was for me. "Sister, Father Freddy was there in the hospital? Thank you. Why?"

There are many mystics in the world, but some are more unusual. I had met her, as a mystic would say, not by chance. I met her the January before I got sick. It was vacation time at college. And Martin was at home recuperating from an operation. Father Freddy, whom I did not know then, had an appointment to visit the nun. The friend who was going to bring him up could not do it. So I agreed to. Father Freddy told me she was famous. "Bishops, cardinals, and important people come for her help. To get an appointment to visit her can take a year. I'm lucky."

I was interested, with a large grain of salt. While Freddy had his visit, I was invited to have lunch with the chaplain. Then, as it happened, someone came and asked me to join Freddy.

A pleasant, happy woman behind the grill, Sister chitchatted with me for a moment and then continued talking to Freddy. I sat there and distinctly felt that she was communicating to me, silently, while also normally talking straight to Freddy. I definitely felt that she was "talking" to me about my family, and my work, and my problems.

I had never felt like that before. After five or six minutes I broke into the other conversation. "What's happening?" I asked. "Really, what's happening?"

Sister smiled, told me it wasn't important, and to relax. The double communication continued. Then Sister said, "Freddy, I want to talk to April privately. She has such wonderful names for her children." And of course she named them all.

Whatever one feels about mystics, one is at least interested. I felt very safe with her in the past, and much more so after aphasia.

On the phone, she told me to be quiet, and just listen. Her words to me are gone. But the gist of her call was to reassure me of the closeness of Jesus. She was telling me not to be afraid. She was talking of self-abandonment to the Lord, and letting Him take over. She promised me that soon someone would quench my fear of blasphemy and of being crazy.

"Then you know?" I said. "Why Babel?"

Listening to her I could only end up saying, "Thank ya! Thank ya! Thank ya!" I could get back to doing my speech homework and riding my stationary bicycle.

With Mary Ball I was slowly learning to figure out how to understand the television. Like a three-year-old I had sort of an idea of the people talking. Partly it was like being deaf—watching and wondering. For me there was sound without meaning. I could concentrate for about four or five minutes, and then the brain dropped into a shell.

It was more fun resting from physical and mental exercising and just seeing life. Next to the playroom, the warmth of the sun sheltered the french pussy willows. "The pussies are moving," I said to Mary Ball.

"No. They're not moving. It's a different word you need. Tell more of what you want to say."

"Today they're not the same. They're a little bigger."

"Growing?"

"O.K.! Growing. Look at it. Look at it. Always look at growing." I saw the birches, and the oak, moving in the wind. "The trees are growing."

Ben Cariri was also trying to explain to me that time sequence changes the language.

I said, "When I was a child I loved using big words. They *sound* nice. I'm a show-off. But so much I want to say."

"Keep telling me what you see," said Ben. "I won't always change your words. Tenses don't matter yet. Talk it out and try the words."

"When I see God's words, I hold part of it with loveliness. I see the tree. It is growing. Every day it changes. I see growing and I see better because I have time to see it and listen. He made it. Do you see it?"

A good speech teacher, Ben told me of spring coming and of the ideas of months.

"The word is January now," I said.

"No, the month is January. Can you name the months?"

Slowly the words were being put together. Try to name trees, birds, fruits, the names of cars. Make a notebook and try to remember them. Say the numbers. Say your number. By rote I learned. I remembered teaching my children: "Where do you live? If you were lost, where would you go and what would you do? Ask the policeman."

Damn it! I had to do the same thing.

To Ben I said, "Teach me that damn word God gave me . . . HEWM———."

Humility was the word, and I couldn't finish it. It was two more years before I could say it. *HEWM!* I used that unfinished word constantly and hardly anyone knew what I was talking about.


When Father George Maloney came to my house, he knew what the word meant, spoken and unspoken. What joy when he came for a whole day! The pussy willows were light gray and singing in the slow rain outside the playroom, and he saw them.

I had come to know him at Fordham, taking a course with him, and visiting him in the John XXIII Building of the Eastern Rite. In one course I had studied of Palamas and the Hesychasts, and had come to learn much from Maloney, a man of spiritual discipline and deep mysticism. Maloney had been one of the mentors on my dissertation, for the twentieth-century Anglican theologians bridge St. Augustine and the Trinity in the Eastern writers of the past. During the summer of 1972, I had tried to write a chapter on the new book and asked him for his opinion. He told me I was on the right track but almost off it, too. He was right. My brain had been about ready to break!

Yet now we talked for hours. And Babel was suspended. I told Father everything that had occurred. I told him that I was afraid. "Could it be that I am sick not from the aneurysm but from the work of the devil? Could I be making it all up, to pretend, to show off? Isn't it possible that, when I lost all my marbles in this aphasia, that my sick mind had produced real mental illness worse than any? If so, absolve me!"

"You couldn't tell a lie if you wanted to," said Father. "Nor are you mentally ill. You have a religious dis-ease. Ease is being lazy. Religious dis-ease is a readiness, an alertness for God's commands."

I sighed with relief. "But I remember Teresa, and John of the Cross, and so many others. I never heard of a so-called mystic that couldn't communicate well, or read, or write, or whatever."

"St. Caedmon, the first English poet, couldn't read or write either. April, who knows what is ahead? But this I know: You are quite clear. You make perfect sense. And you must never be afraid. You are truthful."

Ben had said my assignment was to go to the supermarket with Mary Ball and shop. I'd "read" the newspaper, look at an ad. Please note: the word was *ads*. What a difference there is in learning to spell. The sound is the same in *ad* and *add*. But when one is a child, or an aphasic, the confusion is awful. Learning the words and seeing them is one thing. But remembering what the sound is, and translating them?

"Have you seen this ad?"

I'd think: I have done my adding for the day, and I had not been doing well with 7+3. To add is hard. All the 7's seemed to get lost in my brain.

"I saw the add and it was pretty bad." But, looking at Mary, I'd understand she meant something else and quite often I'd get darn' cross.

But when we went over to Palmer's supermarket I would get so excited staring at things, I'd forget what we came for. No wonder tots are sure it's an amazing place. Tots sit in shopping carts. I, like other disabled people, find them sturdy; you can rest by partly balancing over them. And then we see and smell and feel things others take for granted. Go close to the place where milk, cheese, and eggs are. There are coldness and strange textures. Like any other child, I decided the colors of plastic pinks and greens over eggs were pretty but squooshy, and the cardboard ones felt more real.

Mary had finished the shopping and found me studying Wesson oil.

"Some are round. And some are sort of turned in and out. Why?"

Poor Mary, but I was learning a large vocabulary. "How do you open things?" I asked. As nearly as I could see, the incision in my head had sliced through all lines of mechanical actions. To turn things? Turn on and off? Close doors and open them, and jars and gadgets? (Five years later, I finally almost learned the difference between *push* and *pull*.)

To be able to take care of myself during the day, I had a lot to learn. Mary and I had agreed that it was time to not have a baby sitter for me. At least Mary agreed, and intellectually I agreed too. But inside myself I couldn't really mean it. I set a date, hesitating.

"Next month I'll be alone all day," I said bravely. "What month will that be?"

"April, the month will be February."

Oh, well, children are very smart, and very much in need of security. Honestly, I couldn't remember perfectly the months of the year. February was hard to say. But I also didn't want Mary to leave me, and I partly pretended. Tots can be sneaky, but they are also asking for help on a deeper level, and they're so simple that they can't lie well. Aphasics, like children, are acting out, forgetting the words they need, calling themselves helpless. It takes a good therapist to help them be firm, and yet fill them with confidence.

Ornery is the word for me, anyway. But I began to learn more about Babel. Aphasics are contrary because they need help completely from others, and only the love of non-aphasics can teach them.

"I love you," said Mary Ball. "And before February is through you'll swing it."

So we went home and I had a long sleep, and then we went back to Palmer's to go over a list of ads.

By then I could walk around quite well, and at least I could finally go to Mass.

The first months at home, I had the joy occasionally of communion with Father Al Watts. Martin had sent away for a beautiful missal for the homebound, so I could follow the Mass on Channel 11. With that and with the Jewish hour on Fridays

on the radio, and the Sunday-night prayers from Father Al
Sienkiewicz, I felt nourished. But I was always waiting, hop-
ing, for the time when I could be with Martin in the church of
St. Cecilia, together with others, in a community of Christian
fellowship. The dream and the reality were quite different, and
I had much to learn about.

I had wanted to get friends to help me to learn my prayers. I
had wanted them to show me how to spell "Halloween." One
or two tried, and meant to again, but as mothers they had so
many things to do for their own children. Catechists are for
children, and their work is difficult. But I do believe that
parishes must become more aware of the special needs of
stroke victims, especially in the first few months. Like Father
Al Watts having Mass for the senile, we need to remember the
prisoners of Babel.

I needed a thread pulling me back to community life. What
is a bishop? What is penance? Ben Cariri had at least given me
a list of words that were part of my life. I looked at them, and
put them in my folder. Oh, God, there are so many words to be
learned! And I could not even know the word "saint," let alone
"Francis" and "Anthony." When friends would stop by, I fre-
quently showed them a large wooden statue that was a special
gift from the students at Sacred Heart. The statue had been
through a fire. One side was deeply charred, while the other
remained its light, natural-wood color. I had placed it in the
nearby wood, next to a birch tree.

"Tell me again how to say it?"

But my frustration drove me crazy, and people would think
of me as quite churly, and sick in the head. I hadn't learned
how to translate my thoughts into words when I got angry.

But I had believed, after a while, that when I went to
church, then people would accept me into "the communion of
saints." Only, they didn't. They had not been taught the mean-

ing of the words "communion of saints." People nodded very kindly, but austerely. I had forgotten the changes in the liturgy. The Church was slowly teaching it. By "law" people were told to shake hands in giving the sign of peace. On the television it seemed they did really give Christ's peace to all. But the peace of the Lord at St. Cecilia's was more like a nervous "How do you do."

I was a child this time, and I saw things clearly. I wanted to stand up in the middle of church and say: "Hey! Don't be in such a rush! This is the Lord's day. Let us rejoice and be glad in it. You're too uptight."

But I didn't say it out loud. They are such good people. *Mea culpa!*

Children and the sick show their anger. As a mother, I had always told my children to control their feelings and grow up. Part of my sickness was frustration. Love from others can calm us. But when adults, whether sick or well, are afraid and hurt, the language of Babel takes over. Only by prayer can the hurt be translated.

At the end of February, Mary Ball was finally free and able to do what she wanted to do. If I got scared I could call her. If I had to go to the doctor, she'd come running, and Peg Mooney set up a schedule of good people who would take me to and from speech therapy. How beautiful people are! Some were from our church. But all were real saints.

March was, for me, on decent days, a total wonder of life. I'd walk around the soggy grass watching the crocuses, the squill, breaking up through the mucky dead leaves. I would see them and sing loudly, because the wind made the sound blow away.

And then I noticed dirt. I had not really looked at dirt for years. I walked to the end of the driveway. Where the asphalt ends, I marveled at the colors of black, gray, brown. I didn't know their names then. But I sat down and felt them. There was sand, which came through the car tracks in the snow. A color like light toast, and one like burnt toast, and one from the sea.

Without words! The color brown? What a bore when you learn that word in school. But, as a real child, you could tell its colors of coffee, chocolate, mahogany, red squirrel, oak nut, tan, rust. You knew then, without words, gray cinders, pepper-and-salt, slate, stone at the end of the road. But when you went to school, you didn't have a large vocabulary, so you might have just quit experiencing colors, the basic joy.

"Very interesting!" I would say out loud, because I was being taught some slang. "Very interesting!" was supposed to be funny.

Like any child, you see a color and in your mind match it with something you have seen. Some dirt looked like mashed potatoes, and some like fried potatoes, and some like hashed potatoes.

Oh, God, what fun!

I was smart enough to pretend to be digging in a part of the garden. But I made mud pies, and loved it. I would sit and look up through the budding birches and on up to the clouds. Forty-three years ago, I had seen it this way. I could clearly remember how I felt on the West Side of New York. But this time I was lucky, because this time I could insist on remembering the glory of life, and besides, in New York I couldn't make mud pies.

May and June brought the prodigal incense of viburnum, the daffodils, the hyacinth. I was drunk with life. The mixed-up mind of my brain was not doing well in English, but in Latin I was singing charmingly. My writing was fantastic!

"Regina Chili let tar a way, Alleluia.
Queya quer meruisti part tar way.
Alleluia Resurrectis si cut dixles
Alleluia Oral pro nobis deum Alleluia!"

I wrote them beautifully, but there was a word I couldn't remember. I called some priests, but many had forgotten their Latin. I called Father Botton. He would know and tell me over the phone, and then I could go singing it out for the world to know. And Father took the time to help me.

Clare was home for the summer, and Fulton. Jo and Bill Moran came to visit me. By then I was swimming daily in the Italian Center, doing laps, and that was more fun than my stationary bike.

Knowing that it was almost time for a checkup with Dr. Ray, I was working hard to learn his tests. Ben worked with me too, but he knew better than I. The words I learned were not really grooved into my brain.

Dr. Ray was delighted. I walked well, went swimming, and kept up with my homework.

"Did you play bridge yet?"

"No. But we played five hundred!"

"Have you thought about makeup?"

"I don't think I need it. Especially swimming." The fact was I had no idea how to put it on.

Then out came his quiz.

"Can you name them?"

"A quarter, a dime, a nickel. A penny." I was being careful. "Wubba band." I knew I hadn't said it well, and I got tense.

Dr. Ray changed the subject. "Can you name your address and phone number?"

I smiled, and got an A. "Please tell me about my eyes. I

don't know why, but my left eye is mixed up. I think it's a bit better, but—"

"What scares you?"

"I can get along, but when I go to Mass and I look at the Host there's a quarter of it gone. A void. Why? Will it ever come back?"

He drew me a picture of two eyes, left and right. "God made the eyes in fascinating ways. Perhaps to give you extra strength in case you got hit from the outside. Your front eyes are fine. So, too, is your back. But inside your head there are pieces confused. We'll see. It might come back."

"Will I get all the way back to where I ought to be?"

"Let's see you in six months."

"Dr. Ray, thank you anyway."

I still couldn't say everything.

By now, in New York City, I could walk several blocks. How charming it was to realize that in the fifties everything was straight, numbered by streets, and changed so that all the streets were one-way. I felt safe. Martin's office was at 30 Rockefeller Plaza. I had his telephone number in my purse. And I could go out by myself to St. Pat's.

Just before noon, I was sitting in a pew in silence. Suddenly I remembered a book: *Worlds in Collision,* by Velikovsky. I remembered my father's interest in the book, a study of the Old Testament. Velikovsky believed that the planets and the meteorites did stop the world, not only in Palestine but all over the world when Joshua fought the battle of Jericho. He attested that when the world started again, the magnetic field of the earth was a bit off the track. The North Star was no longer straight north.

At the same time, I felt as if I were in a huge subway that was horribly shaking. I felt the world was in darkness, darkness and ashes for two days and two nights. And then I felt as if the world began to turn, with a whimper, and I felt the earth was going not from east to west but from west to east.

In the darkness people would be afraid. Many would die with fright. Many would run to churches and synagogues, praying, calling out in fear. But soon, too soon, in the light, many again forgot about God. The darkness makes people tremble. But in the light they boast again. See? they would say, we made it.

I felt there was a reason why we would not be able to drink regular water for a while. And I felt I must keep a gallon of regular water with a top on it in the pantry.

At that moment the priest entered and noon Mass began, and I completely forgot about it. But, that night, as I went to sleep in the hotel, I remembered the world in darkness with a strange feeling, and I told Martin and then went right to sleep.

Was that a special vision? Hell, no! Was that a communication from the Lord? Oh, no! Did Jesus say so? In a way, to all people who have read the Bible and meditated on it. There is nothing new, only the truth.

Whenever I go back to St. Pat's, I feel the same feeling. My feeling reminding me that under the stupid nonsense of daily business there is an exploding truth: God. But one does not need a "light" or a "vision." One does not run around knocking on the doors of bishops or popes saying: Hey, I've seen something. One only needs to pray, and share the wonders of the Trinity.

During the summer, I had two quiet quests: makeup and going up to Regina Laudis, to the cloistered Benedictine nuns in Bethlehem, Connecticut. Martin and I went there to see Mother Placid, the most unplacid, vivacious artist and sculptress. She had been my friend for some twenty years and a woman of my age who years before had gently begun teaching me wisdom and compassion. A retreat at Regina Laudis, unstructured, unmolested by talks, renews people with woods, mountains, wholesome food, and benedictional work in the land.

On my night table was the prayer teaching the closeness of Him who waits. To Mother Placid, I told the joy of that prayer: *Suscipe*. We talked of P.T. and speech therapy, frustration and laughter. And I told her about death and life, Jesus and Mary, and my concern about storing water. Poor Mother! when I got excited, my words would get all mumbled around "HEWM!" as I tried to explain to her the unspoken word for humility.

She also suggested that I get some makeup.

"I tried it at home," I said. "I have lots of it in my drawer. And guess what happened? I put blue on my mouth and red on my eyes. It was pretty, but I gathered it was wrong. So I washed it off. I tried it five times and gave up."

"Go to the department store and ask for help," she said. "HEWM, dear."

I chortled. I knew I was "home" with her.

When I arrived home from Regina Laudis, I went to Bloomingdale's in Stamford. I would do as Mother Placid suggested. But I shied away from the cosmetics counters. Salesmen wanted to know what I wanted. My words stumbled. And I moved into other groups, studying all the stuff to be bought. I was too afraid. And I had too much pride. I bought a lipstick and went home. I didn't even need a shower cap yet. My hair was a long crew cut.

For the first seven months after the operation, the sense of smell was gone. Nothing had taste at all. The olfactory sense depends on the nerves at the base of the skull. Anosmia can happen for many reasons. All I know is that I couldn't tell whether the meal was good or whether I needed salt.

Martin and I used to joke about it. I would say, "Having cooked for nine people, I'm delighted not to have to cook anymore. Twenty-five years is long enough. And believe me: I won't even try."

But inside me it wasn't a joke.

During the winter it was still very hard for me to see things close up. I'd sit with Mary Ball in the kitchen while she told me the names of such things as garlic, oregano, and basil. Then I would go to the cabinet and pick up the herb or spice. All cooks have their own special ideas. I liked nutmeg with string-beans. But some I couldn't remember, and I only partly learned to read. As spring came, making my own sandwich I would experiment. I knew there was something I liked to put together with tunafish. I didn't want mayonnaise, because it is fattening. Once, I tried curry. Another day, I tried dill. By the third week I remembered it was mustard. But by then I was contented with peanut butter instead of mustard.

Almost a year had passed. Martin had a vegetable patch outside the house. On a warm afternoon he brought in string-beans. How beautiful they were! The color was cool blue-green. Vegetables are every bit as amazing as flowers. Praise the Lord! Growth, touched by sun. They have a deeply quiet dance, alive.

Martin went out to weed the patch. I coolly washed the stringbeans in his basket. It didn't look right. How do you wash them, I wondered. I looked again under the sink. I couldn't remember the name of the big round thing with holes. (A year later, I could say *colander*.) I found it, then washed the sea-colored vegetables again with running water. How slender a stringbean is, yet what strength it has.

I meditated.

Part of the stuff in the colander looked a little messy. There had been some very rainy days. They should be cleaned up properly, I thought. I looked around. My brain knew. My brain showed me a time when the Fuller Brush lady had come and given me a new brush. I unwrapped it, and began to "give them a bath" of cold water. The dirt went down in the sink. Then the beans looked happy. I sat down to rest, and had some iced coffee.

How, I wondered, do you cook stringbeans? Part of me laughing about not wanting to know how to cook. Another part wanted to help Martin. And another part said, Let's go, kid—there's work to be done.

I looked in the kitchen drawer. Part of the vegetables had to be cut. I tried using my fingers. The beans broke and made nice noises, but I didn't know what to do with the ends? I looked for a knife. An hour later, I was done. I was tired. I gauged the right-size pot, then I called Mary Ball. "How much water would I put in to cook stringbeans?"

God bless her! She said, "April, how great! You are trying to cook!"

Praise is what aphasics need. So I felt good. "Put a little water in the pot. Not lots. Just a little," advised Mary.

"Do you put hot water in, or cold?" Part of me felt so stupid even to ask such questions. But the other part of the brain said, "Ask every question, first."

I put the stringbeans into the pot with cold water, without a lid, and cooked them for about five minutes. Then I put the lid on and boiled the beans at medium.

Like a kid, I kept opening the pot and watching. But soon the water began to go away.

I called Mary again on the telephone. "Do you put more water in?"

So I learned how quickly things are done, and began learning about salt and pepper, butter, and nutmeg.

Martin came in and we were both excited. After two hours we had a vegetable that he had planted and hoed and petted and cut and I had cooked!

Summer was a real gift, the healing part of aphasia. I was still having trouble reading. I had problems seeing, and co-ordinating my body. But, that Christmas, Fulton had given me a fresh copy of the *Good Housekeeping Cookbook*, and it became my homework and my bible. I could read no more than five minutes at a time, then take a break, and read a bit more. There were pictures that would help me understand.

I'd sit and study "short ribs" and "boned rolled rump." I would look at "measuring" and slowly I gathered the notion of cubes. Three-dimensional ideas were very difficult for me.

Unfortunately, this book did not have pictures of everything. So *The American Heritage Dictionary* also lived in my kitchen. I could finally see what a "parsnip" was with that book. But a "paring knife"? No picture.

I would look in the kitchen drawer and wonder what would work to take the top off an apple without using the knife.

I'd call Mary Ball.

"What does it look like, that takes the top off the apples lightly?"

Mary laughed. "I can't remember the name. It's a—you know?"

"Well," I'd say, "if I wanted to get ready to cook a big Rome apple, what would I use?"

"Mmmm . . . ," would say Mary. "It's round and it's uh, gee . . . I can't remember. You know?"

A lot of normal people forget words too. But aphasics are deeply frustrated. Aphasics need complete pictures of things, and want the dignity to not have to ask. I wanted to make mashed potatoes. No picture; I had to call Mary again.

"I know I'm a pain calling you, but what is that thing that you put cooked potatoes into to make them squidgy?"

"I have no idea, April."

"O.K., I'll start from the beginning. The white potatoes are cleaned. Then they are pared. Then they are cooked. I want to put them into a machine, and they will come out the bottom. Then I will add butter and salt. But what's that thing in the middle?"

"A ricer. Or a sieve."

"No, I'm not making rice. I'm making hot potatoes."

"Then put them into the electric mixer. Or use a hand beater."

A communication breakdown. With aphasics the brain is still weak. My brain fell apart; the connections were broken because the word "rice" confused me. The word rice got into the brain computer. Normal people move quickly in their brain, offering many ideas. Electric mixer and rice? I wanted to cry!

I found two big round things. One was a sieve. Another was a colander. I tried both. The potatoes were already pretty cold. I wept. Then I put the potatoes into a double boiler with water, and said I didn't care for mashed potatoes anyway.

The aphasic needs confidence, and cooking is a wonderful gift for returning to life. The disabled needs exercising and therapy. But even more he needs dignity, and a purpose, challenging and real. Everybody is hungry, every day. And then there is the human hunger for doing a worthwhile job.

Relearning to cook, I wondered at the glory of colors in the vegetable. I would buy a box of mushrooms and marvel at them. What color are they? Fresh, clean, they are the color of unopened eggs next to the earth, off-white and brown.

A green pepper? So dark emerald, yet not so shiny, a bit sexy. Open it with a paring knife and see the egg-white softness inside the pepper.

Oh, eggplant! Deepest amethyst, so dark it seems illuminated purple, touched with olive green at the tip. Beautiful!

But also confusing. The mind of the aphasic is swimming with confusion. What is the difference between an unopened egg, egg whites, and eggplant? Speech teacher, where are you?

Thank God, there was Ben around.

I believed there was a need for a special book on cooking for aphasics. I had been a writer and had sold a few articles to *Good Housekeeping*. So I wrote a letter and sent a manuscript. I said I cannot write as I used to. The words get mixed up. There's no grammar. There's no sense. But could you realize the need to help others, to add to your cookbook? Politely, I got a rejection. But time passes. I still believe aphasics need a cookbook with colored pictures of meat and vegetables and fruit.

Meanwhile I was cooking, and making gorgeous mistakes. Paul was having a party, and with greatest joy, I made my special recipe of spaghetti casserole. I had done it almost by rote, and I also reread it over and over. It looked beautiful. But even our dogs couldn't eat it. I had not learned the difference between tablespoons and teaspoons. Three tablespoons of salt was a bit heavy.

And yet . . .

By that time, I was learning to write. I could spell the phrase: "and yet. . . ." The more I learned, the more I saw my situation. A two-year-old isn't concerned about the future. But a second-grade kid knows if his speech is different from others. I was by then the equivalent of a slightly retarded child. One of the important tests for a child is to see if he can understand a joke. I could not see what was funny in anything.

My wonderful friends bringing me to speech therapy had young children.

"Tell me your jokes?" I would ask. Ben Cariri had told me I needed to understand.

"What's black and white and read all over?" one chanted happily. Or another would say, "Idaho; Alaska."

I didn't know what they were talking about. The kids had whole books of jokes, and they laughed. I was smart enough to know that that meant I was really stupid.

Parts of my brain were mending. I would suddenly understand what furniture polish was for. And I would polish every piece of wood in our house, and do a good job. But I could not understand anything about silver polish. Everything in my mind was separated. Ben's picture of library cards fallen on the floor was true. I could understand all about polishing wood. But my brain could not associate that with other stuff to clean other things.

I was in Ben's waiting room. "Oh, God, I'm stupid," I said.

"No. You're awfully angry, though," Jesus said.

"Yes," I said.

"Look what I have done to you," He said. "I have given you a gift."

I said nothing but "Why?" Then I remembered my prayer. *Suscipe.*

"I gave it to you freely," He said.

"But why?"

In the waiting room was a child about four years old, a real pain in the rump. But I looked in his eyes for a moment, and I saw him. He was a prisoner of language problems. He knew the anger and the horror of "normal" life.

"Lord, are You in this child now?"

"I am," He said. "I am in every child. I am a prisoner. This child sees the truth. It is not pretty. It is awesome."

"My God," I said very quietly. "Why?"

"Look truthfully at your cross. And his."

After a few moments I asked: "Why? What is the point?"

"You are not ready to understand. My Word is not with words. You cannot speak it. But you must sing it. Sing the unspoken. Sing joyfully, sing sadly, sing out of the depths. Sing in Bethlehem and sing on the cross. Sing human. Praise and sing."

O.K. Flat and off key, or right on key, the unknown meaning of my life was in bondage, singing for someone else to set me free. Penance? Possible. For the dyslexics, for the retarded, for the aphasics, for the senile, there is a yoke. But we also have the gift of seeing the truth.

Mary Walsh went regularly to the convalescent homes, running an hour of the rosary. She was kind to bring me with her. I, who love great Mary, Mother of Jesus, could not manage a long rosary. But I could see the truth in those around us.

One woman constantly spoke with nasty curses. I understood that part of Babel. Another woman said nothing. Her language muted, she cried and cried and cried. In their faces I saw His truth.

To one I said, "No wonder you're crying."

Of another I asked, "How hungry are you?" The blind helping the blind, translation in Babel. She wanted so much to go to communion.

"Yes, Goddam it." She spitted out her words, and grabbed at my hand.

Someone, noticing my stupid words and hers, brought her a tray of cookies. She threw them on the floor.

I spoke with a priest deeply involved in ministering to the

senile. I realized priests' awful responsibility with the sick. But in my way I do not care how one classifies people. Demons? Religiously or psychologically? The New Testament said only: Do you know who I am? I have come to visit the sick, break the bonds.

The learned people insist that aphasics are not on the same level as the senile or the retarded. "It's partly a matter of IQ," they say. "And a physical difference when the brain is damaged."

"We're all in the same boat," I'd say. "Don't classify us. Just heal us in your own way. But translate with love."

People were as kind to me as they could be. Clergymen, doctors, therapists, all agreed I was wrong. And on one level, they're right and I'm wrong. Clinically, there is a real difference between senility and aphasia. But, from the other side of Babel, I see a certain kind of truth.

Good people, kind people, fall into dangerous religious games. And the devil himself leads many of them on a merry-go-round of "piety." Visiting the sick is fine. But praying for a miracle? God save us from that. Some come to the unhealed, in hospitals and at home, hoping to heal without treading gently on the holy. And sometimes they do more harm than good. Do you remember the story of the paralytic whose friends brought him to be healed by Jesus? He healed the man's sins. But who wanted that? Their friends, used to that merry-go-round of piety, begged for Jesus to heal him physically. He did it. But I have often wondered how the healed man felt, carrying away his paralytic bed on his back.

I was not totally healed. I had so much to learn, slowly.

I remember another afternoon in August. Chris Golightly and Martin and I were sitting on the grass. Sometimes I talked well, but so many people kept remarking sadly that I was not at all the way I used to be. Martin was lonely. I was watching the robin next to the sprinkler, and looking at the color of dark green and earth and earthworm pink.

She looked in my eyes. "I see her," she said. "God has his own meaning."

I heard her. "This is the day the Lord has made," I sang. "And it's also your birthday. I made a cake for you."

What would we do without friends? Thank goodness the cake I made for her was edible, even though the frosting was out of kilter.

My quest on makeup?

I had tried to get help at department stores, pharmacies, and discount places. I'd browse and study commercials. I'd look in my bathroom at all the stuff I had and try to figure it all out. After all, I was pretty smart at finally learning to brush my teeth. At my age I ought to figure out what "eyelashes" mean by looking in the dictionary. I'd end up with mistakes. I'd put on remover cream and pat brown color over it.

Oh, well! The time came when Martin and I were going to stay in a hotel in Manhattan, with dinner and theater, and so I took all the makeup I owned, put it in a tote bag, and walked into Bergdorf Goodman's.

I, who never normally shopped there, walked over to the kindest-looking saleswoman who wasn't busy and said, "I need help. I have aphasia. I know nothing. Here is everything I used to use. Can you teach me? Tell me what to do from waking up in the morning till I go to sleep at night."

She looked in my bag. "Most of it, you already have. Great!" Over in a corner she gently taught me. "You really don't know basic words? But you've got spunk."

"I've got a wonderful speech pathologist, but that's not his line."

After one hour I thought I looked pretty good. The bill was only thirty-five dollars.

"Now," she said. "Go home to the hotel. Take off all your makeup. And start over. Then come on back and show me. You'll feel safe."

Two hours later, I came back.

"Well done!" she said. "Now I want to tell you something: You have to push yourself up. Some people may say, who do you think you are? Forget them. Think of yourself. Who do you think you are? Worthwhile!"

Oh, I felt good. What a woman! A month later, I stopped by to thank her again, but she came running toward me.

"Your wonderful husband wrote a letter to Mr. Goodman. I was called up to his office. I never heard of such a thing. Your husband is unusual, so kind."

I agreed.

But I still felt unsure about everything in the normal world. I felt safe at Kropotkin's. I felt safe at Bergdorf's. I heard two of my friends talking about me.

"At least she's learned how to manage money. She's not buying clothes there. But she has lunch there sometimes."

"And she buys hats at thrift shops. I can't understand her."

"Neither do I," I said, "but I love New York City."

Only later would I begin to understand why.

But then I only knew that from the forties to the seventies all the streets were safe, with one-way streets, and numbers, not words. I could stop by St. Pat's, window-shop, and have lunch with Martin. In the city I felt safe, unnoticed in the crowd, where I could wonder at life. Museums, bagel carts, dime stores, Tiffany's. I learned the better places for the ladies' rooms; I learned that one can walk and sing and nobody's shocked and many sing with you. I felt free as a hermit, eccentric but unknown.

I didn't talk much to others. Seeing was enough, until the time came when I absolutely had to find a language. I needed some health equipment immediately. I ran into the nearest pharmacy. But I couldn't find it on the counter. I really could not remember the word of what I wanted.

I walked out, terrified. I went back again. And I walked out again. No language.

*Learn to translate.*

In the fifties there were many signs: French spoken. German spoken. Spanish spoken. I couldn't pretend: Aphasia spoken here.

I was standing on Fifty-eighth Street on the West Side, where a wonderful old character actress lived. She had taught my mother to act on stage. *Thanks, Mom!* I went back to the pharmacy.

"English I not speak well yet. Croat Yugoslav. I'm trying. Can you help me? Can I look back there for what I want? Then you can tell me the name."

Back in the hotel I pondered. I'm not a very good actress, but I like being a fool. It's more fun. I hated asking for help. I had lost all that dignity and confidence, but I still had tons of pride. Was it pride that sent me to a swanky store? Was it pride that brought me to that unusual gift store? Couldn't I have gone somewhere else? Until all my mind returned, I knew I still had to play a game. I could not drop pride in myself.

So I played the game beautifully whenever I was in New York. Sometimes I pretended I was Hungarian, as long as I wasn't on the East Side. Once I even used Swahili. With any language, one needed only a phrase to pretend. Through Father John de Marchi I had learned, "In the name of the Father, the Son, and the Holy Spirit," in Swahili. It sounded nice.

Of course, I had not reached the abstract level of language. It had never occurred to me that few white people were born learning Swahili.

Someone did ask me.

"Swahili from the South," I said, bursting out with laughter. Babel translates. Pride falls down.

The winter came with winds, the ice, the finches, and homework. I spoke better. I could read a bit. Pride slaughtered me. Ben gave me a children's version of *Reader's Digest*.

"My dad? My brother? Don't you know the damn *Reader's Digest* is part of our life? I won't read this!"

And I nearly cried. But truthfully the *Digest* was the best reader for me. There would be a short story and questions to be answered.

Aphasia is a disease designed to drop pride and help a person see truth, at least for me.

In December the year was up. During my checkup, Dr. Ray for the first time talked only with me.

Do you remember bringing a child to the doctor? Do you remember when the kid grew up enough to talk to the doctor without Mom around? A really big deal! Martin had to wait outside, in the office. My brain was healed enough to communicate well.

I watched the doctor's eyes. He's a brisk man, abrupt, leveling with real love. "That's about as far as you're going to go. Can you take it?"

"You mean you really don't think I'll ever get back to writing or teaching?"

"It doesn't look like it."

I was proud of him. I thanked God for him. He was evaluating my "condition." He had noticed that I could now name paper clips. I could count down from one hundred to fifty, but my sevens were off. There was no great change in my "condition."

"April, your eyes are better, and I think you can drive again, though not in traffic. You made a good comeback."

I wanted to scream. "I want to thank you," I said. "I would have been happier if I could have stayed in heaven. But I was sent back. Your job was to fix me. And I was sent back like a turkey that was undercooked. There was a reason why I wasn't ready. But most of all, I bless you for putting things on the table for me and telling me where I stand. I love you. But maybe you're wrong."

"See you in June, April. Who knows?"

I went to St. Pat's and hid myself in a corner.

He was there.

## CHAPTER SIX

Holidays are bleak for those not ready to look at truth.

Thanksgiving and Christmas are times to call and visit. I found them frustrating. I was lonely, and I was glad to see anybody anytime, but I also really wanted to be nasty and sarcastic.

"Where were you the rest of the year? Why not spread out your payments of love over other months?" I thought it but didn't say it. I was trying to learn humility, and botching it.

Thanksgiving confused me. I had never really understood the deep question of helping the poor through the churches. Isn't it right and pleasing to bring a turkey to the unemployed, the sick, the down and out? Yes. The good mean well, as I had done too in the past. I realized that the poor had a more difficult cross to bear: to accept alms.

I knew of a woman who received three turkeys with all the fixings. She felt like throwing one in the faces of the club that brought it, an unwanted kind gift. Her pride accepted it sardonically, and made a joke of it, passing it on to others. Where were we in January, May, August? Busy elsewhere, meaning well but busy. Moneywise, I had never been poor. But I was poor, afflicted. So, too, were my family.

Friends would call on me in the holidays, and quite soon I would say something crotchety like "Oh, what a bore!"

I wonder what similar words come out of the afflicted.

Another phrase of mine was "Grow up!"

Only now my family tell me how awful it was, hearing me

say that. They cringed to see me coming, sure that I would say the same things over again. Most of the time, those words did not stick in my mind at all. Yet occasionally I would hear myself, and as a prisoner I would ask myself why.

Why do you give such a horrible cross to others?

I clearly remember a day when a close friend, a godly priest, John, greeted me with real love. I almost started to cry. I wanted to hold him so close. Instead, with a big smile I said clearly, "Oh, what a bore!"

What horror! I didn't know why. I felt badly, but I couldn't say anything. I was stuck.

And for two more years, I wondered. I would hear myself in my mind and ask *why?*

Then, in 1977, the same thing occurred. There was a communication break, untranslated Babel that I heard coming from myself. My daughter and I have a good relationship. But something happened and our wave lengths were miles apart. I talked, she talked, I explained, she explained, I knew, she knew—impasse. No rapport. I wanted to scream and pull out my hair. But studying magazine psychology, I said we should stop talking for a while, and withdraw.

"We'll talk about it another time," I said. And I hung up the phone and said, "Oh, what a bore!"

I would have sworn that, so as not to hurt her, I said it only after hanging up. But my unconscious level said it so she could hear it.

Quite quickly we were friends again. But my daughter told me what I'd said. What real joy! For the first time in five years, I understood the tongue of Babel.

Translation: What a bore! means: Woe!!!

It is a cry, a wail, smothered. One swallows the cry of the cross. The wail wants to come out and scream: O my God, I need You! Help!

But, partly feeling ashamed and partly not wanting to intrude on others, one puts on a garment to cover the cry. And the unconscious without translation tells the truth.

What a bore, most of the holidays mean. I needed a deep, deep hug, not a toast. And I wasn't strong enough to give a hug to others.

"We're not talking right," I said. Caught in pain, the pus of loneliness and fear does not fit with pretense.

"Look in the mirror," said Jesus.

I ran to the mirror. Usually one looks there only when one's deciding to fix oneself up. But this time I caught myself. I saw the anger and hardness in my face.

"You are trying to be nice, but you're not truthful. You look as if you are about to explode," He said.

"I don't want to be."

"Prophets have to suffer."

"I'm not a prophet, Lord; I am a mess."

"All who love My Heart are prophets. They are suffering. Your family is suffering, and your family are prophets. Don't you know that yet? Look across the street. Look at other families: all prophets. Don't you see Me in others? I'm there. My Word is locked in their Babel."

Looking in the mirror again, I almost wanted to break it, to throw it away. "You're telling me I'm a sinner."

"I love sinners."

"But I'm trying to be good! What is goodness? I am not worthy of You, but I'm trying. Why do You let me say things and do things to hurt others? Why do the wrong words come out?"

"Prophets have to live and accept and wait till the code key is broken."

"I hate it. I'm not a prophet."

"You are a servant of Mine."

"A lousy one."

"I agree. But Mine. And I have other servants and I love them. It's time for you to learn: Judge not. Judge no one."

"Yes, Lord."

"Look in the mirror from time to time. See yourself. And feel sorry for My other servants who see you. I chose you to be My servant as an example." There was silence, and then He said: "You still are not truthful enough to ask Me why I can't make you or your family or your friends turn perfect. I need salt on the earth."

I stared at the mirror, but I couldn't see it clearly.

"When you translate Babel, keep a glass mirror nearby. 'Oh, what a bore' is a language block. Go tell John. Tell him he's not a bore. Tell him the prophet's swallowed cry, and make every day a holiday."

New Year's Eve with Martin was always a quiet time, looking back over the past year, making wishes and resolutions, followed with special games and betting for pennies on roulette and horses.

Our children had grown, and with joy Chris Golightly came to greet 1974 with us. In September, Paul had decided to try out a high school year in St. Francis' Seminary. Clare was living at home, a sophomore in Stamford Catholic High. Caedmon, Fulton, Cathy, Michael, Marty, how quickly the years pass. To list the wishes and hopes for the New Year always mixes joy, sadness, and a middle ground. Isn't that true for everyone?

Truly, what was my situation? I was able to read, slowly, in the third-grade reader. I could type about five lines before being overwhelmed with frustration. I could not write a decent letter. I could not remember anything about the sciences or the humanities. I could not sew or read music.

"Oh, come on, April! Now list the things you can do," said Chris. "You drove the car to bring Cathy to the hospital."

"Yes. And I was scared to death. They said I could drive if I stayed out of traffic. But I did it."

"You cooked a good dinner. You almost learned how to set the table. You decorated for Advent and Christmas. You signed your own cards."

"Chris! A good minister stopped by to visit me, and I let him study my dissertation. But I don't even know what it was about!"

"So list it. And keep on. You can now walk half a mile. You can . . ."

She is a prophet too. When two or three are gathered together we must tell ourselves. She was filling in the goodness I needed. And the middle part too.

"My wish for the coming year," I said, "is to learn my nursery rhymes." Ben had been telling me to learn them, and I hadn't. Clare had been trying to teach me. "I hate them, but I will. And I wish—" I burst out laughing! "I wish I could really learn *Suscipe*, that darn' prayer, by heart. 'Take, O Lord, all my memory, and my understanding, and my will'; I guess I might have been trying to take it back."

For the New Year I got three wishes.

One was a small change that occurred in my eyes. The Picasso painting feeling disappeared. From my way of seeing it, some of the voids were healing. I could, for example, see some new pieces in the lens. I could see the whole Host at communion. The eye men explained that my peripheral vision was all right, but there were still some voids in my right eye. I could drive, but I had to be careful to turn toward the right side of the car.

A second wish had to do with music.

As a child I had to learn the piano. For this I thank my mother. I was never good, but by playing and studying and singing in a group I found that discipline and joy work together, mingling with the souls of others.

One of my resolutions for the New Year was to relearn music. By memory I could sing, and at the monastery in New Canaan I could sing without upsetting people. I, who had been an alto, was now a very low tenor. At home I could play some songs by rote on the piano, but I could not see all the notes. I, who had taught most of my children how to read notes, could not remember the meaning of do, re, mi, C, D, E. So I bit my tongue and found the very first lessons I had used for Cathy. I had put gold stars on the pages when she learned them.

O.K.! I found that with my aphasia I could read notes, or read the words, or watch my fingers. But I could not do all three at once. To put a finger on middle C and say "C" at the same time was really exhausting. The mechanism of my brain was apparently weak.

I turned on my tape recorder to record my mistakes. I would put my finger on D and sing the right note, but quite often I played and sang the note calling it "B." Patience, I said, and worked for half an hour a day regularly.

Then, one day, I got a call from Joe Rich. He was the manager of quality control in a plastics factory. He was also a choir conductor, a man dedicated to music and the Lord. For many years I had worked under him at St. Cecilia's Church, quitting only with the pressure of finishing my doctoral studies. The first Christmas after the aneurysm, he came to visit me right after Mass. It had touched me deeply, because as he sat with me in the living room he looked as if he would cry.

"When you're stronger, April," he said, "I need you to sing." I hadn't believed him.

But in 1974 he said, "We are now singing regularly at Holy

Spirit Church. Helena would pick you up on Thursday evenings for choir rehearsal. Mass will be Sunday at eleven."

"Oh, come on," I said. "My range is one octave below middle C. I can't read or remember music."

"Oh, shut up! Don't tell me about it. So be a tenor who can't read! Your job is to come."

With his wife, Helena, at the organ, and Joe conducting, many miracles occurred. With the best collection of music from medieval to modern, with love, fortitude, and confidence, the whole choir was alive and aware of God. There was room for me. I would try, and make mistakes. My brain would falter after about half an hour and I would forget where I was.

"When you're tired, sit down. It won't bother us."

I would start crying with frustration by the coffee break.

"We love you as you are," said Joe. "You're doing fine."

What a saint! His words were imprinted in my mind. *We love you as you are.* No faking. No pretending.

Speech pathologists had explained to me that singing was not the same as language skill. Stroke people can sing by rote, they say, but they do not study with it. I am not an expert on this question. But I know that those who sing pray twice. The task of connecting the pieces in my brain was still incomplete. But I believe what deeply healed me was a feeling of being accepted in normal life. Two hours of singing was exhausting and exciting. But I was not cooped up in the house, constantly reminded of my problems.

Helena, who had been praying for my recovery from the time of my illness on; Helena, devoted to St. John Neumann, prayed for me and helped me learn both the tenor and the alto lines.

Joe Rich is in heaven now, no longer taking his angina pills, no longer getting angry at people who would not work as hard as he did to praise the Lord. But much of my recovery came through him.

The third gift for that New Year was actually a parable. Cathy and her child, Ginny, had moved to Stamford. But Cathy was sick. For at least a year, possibly longer, the doctors made it clear, she would not be able to take care of the child. Martin and I set up a crib and paraphernalia with joy, love, and nervousness. Then we called for help! The want ad read:

> Unwell Grandmother caring
> for an almost two-year-old seeks
> babysitter with own transportation
> 9–4 p.m. Monday through Friday in
> Springdale–Newfield area. No other
> duties. Call 322-5113.

Alice Carlheim was not looking for a job. Retired, comfortably situated, she was sitting with her feet up. Tiny, a bit tired, she sipped her coffee and, having read the rest of the paper, she idly looked at the want ads. The Lord had a reason. A grandma with many projects in store, she stared at the ad. Her life was full: with the writing of poetry, with stories of her time in Sweden, with her delight as an interior decorator, and with her Lutheran love of God. Practically, the job seemed difficult at her age. So she called our house. And that was the first link in a beautiful friendship.

Soon we were tooling around the town as Alice taught Ginny and me how to behave in practical matters. I was relearning how to clean, and how to co-ordinate my hands so I would not grab small people and hurt them. Ginny had to be trained to obedience with laughter and hugs. An odd picture we made at Lord and Taylor's for lunch, and browsing through the United Home Wrecking junkyard, singing "Peter, Peter, pumpkin eater," and talking about the Bible. We jelled perfectly. My children had no living grandma. I needed a sister. What a wish granted!

Just as music is necessary for the sick, so, too, is art. The rational part of the brain is starving for communication. I was still looking at the daily newspaper, as Dr. Ray had ordered. I could focus and I could "read," but the brain had not really understood the meaning. Then, suddenly, one day in the New York *Times,* I really read about an art exhibit. The articles on religion, world news, politics, meant nothing to me. But I could suddenly understand stories of art, what I knew in the past and what was relevant today. A couple of times a month, I would encase myself in the Museum of Modern Art, with visits back to the Metropolitan. I was actually hungry for painting and sculpture, the mind drinking deeply. Images on the irrational level of aphasia needed guidance.

At the same time, I began trying to draw and paint. All my life I knew I was not an artist. But I had learned in college that, to understand art, one had to attempt to copy it. The body language needed to get the feeling, to communicate and accept the message of the artist.

With Alice I picked up a child's double easel, paper, colored pencils, and acrylic paint. Ginny could scribble on one side, and I could study on the other. The playroom was a gorgeous mess. My right hand was forced to use discipline in trying to color. Free form, prekindergarten, and finger painting allowed me to be free. But also, unlike Ginny, I needed a feeling of accomplishment. Cards, simply designed, would be useful. Thinking about Easter, I thought of life, death, and resurrection. I thought of our human life as of insect larvae. I thought of death as of a cocoon. I thought of resurrection as of a butterfly at last. For a month I would design the simplest Easter cards I could. The cocoon, I studied from a garden book, and the butterfly on the inside of the card I made larger than life. By Easter I had enough made for all my friends. Beautiful? Intellectually, no. But therapy includes the gentleness of a friend accepting a gift.

And Martin, so kind, bought me a signed lithograph of a painting, by Carolyn Blish, of a child at the edge of the sea.

For the first time in a year and a half, I had a three-day vacation, free from learning my speech homework. I wanted to go on retreat at the Cenacle, in Connecticut. Mary Walsh was also interested, and her daughters drove us up there. There are many ways of running retreats. What we wanted at the time was quietness, little chitchat, but no formal lectures. At meals someone read out loud. A sister was available for studying. A confessional was nearby. And the chapel was always open. Outside there were places to walk, to meditate, in the woods or in the gardens.

The place was wintry, covered with snow, with few people around. I was so beautifully happy! The last time I had been there, I was excitedly studying more of Teilhard de Chardin and the lectures of Ewert Cousins, my mentor. I opened the door to look at the room where Cousins had been speaking, and giggled. I saw clearly the outlines of my two teachers, Teilhard and Cousins, in my mind, but the rational level of the brain was still up in the stars. "Sometimes," I said, "who knows?" and ran out to the brilliant sun. Walking made a crunching sound, and in the shade the white snow was a light purple mist.

Oh, what fun! Here and there were statues crowned with snow. Feeling safe, I began to sing songs to the statues. If nobody is watching you, you can be a child. Alleluia, Sacred Heart!

"Hi, world, *everybody*," I shouted. "How are you?" I passed a small area for St. Joseph, all covered with white. I had never been deeply involved in St. Joseph, but I nodded and went on over the Stations of the Cross. Some I brushed the snow from. Some I did not.

Then, on the way back, I looked again at Joseph, and I knew I was physically tired and needed to sit down. So I dusted the snow from a concrete bench and rested.

"Why don't you think of me?" asked Joseph.

"I've never understood you," I said.

Joseph said, "I always loved God, the Lord. And I did the best for Him as I understood it. But I was always working, and worrying."

"Like so many men? They worry so much."

He nodded.

I got up and cleared the snow from his face and his worker's hands.

"And then, I myself was told about Jesus before He was born."

"I had thought about that. How did you feel?"

"I said, 'Yes, Lord. . . .' But what could I do but worry, and be afraid? Oh, Lord, my God. Who is the Son in my house? Who is the Holy Spirit sending to me? Who, O Lord God, the almighty One? The wonderful One is the Redeemer? My *Child?* My *Brother?* My *King? Alleluia?* The words don't make sense, do they? Even today. But the Word does," Joseph said. "The Father seems so great and so good, but far away from problems. And I was caring and worrying. And then, angels had to put me to sleep to tell me what God wanted done. And I said, 'Yes, Lord. . . .' And what could I do but take Mary to be my wife, the mother of Jesus."

"Oh! You were the father of the house. What would you say?"

"My Child? My Brother? My King?" asked Joseph.

Hesitating, I sang, "Alleluia? Alleluia, O Lord God, Alleluia!"

Joseph said, "My Jesus seemed too great and so small. Far

away I could love Him, but not near—for I was confused and
worried! But then, my Mary and her Son brought me nearer,
to love the Father and our Son. And I said, 'Yes, Lord!' It takes
time to love, to be open and not afraid!" Then he said, "O
Lord, my God, this is the Son in God's house! This is the Holy
Spirit sending strength to us! My Child, my Brother, *my* King!"

"Alleluia."

Joseph said, "I tell you of the love of the Three-in-One. Believe it before you can understand it. Then you'll never be confused or worry. And then I'll tell you about Jesus, the paradox
of God. And I say, 'Yes, Lord'; human and divine meet in this
love, unafraid. This is the love, present in all love! This is the
Holy Spirit mending the love in us! The paradox, the Redeemer: my Child, my Brother, *my* King."

In the rising twilight, the colors were sharply etched in gold
over purple. Like a nut, I wanted to dance all the way back to
the house, but my feet were almost frozen and I fell down and
hobbled home laughing.

"You do seem much better for the vacation," said the priest
as he helped me in. We had been talking before, as he was interested in the problems of aphasia. From a theological perspective he was studying the questions of confession for the
convalescent homes.

"Amazing! Real aphasics," he said, "cannot tell a lie. What a
gift!"

But a coin always has two sides. When I came home from
the retreat, I did feel better, more healed. And within the
week, standing outside of the monastery in New Canaan, talking with Mary Walsh, I said something that was actually a lie.
She had asked me if I had heard a certain theologian giving a
special talk.

"Were you there?"

"I was. What he said was right."

She accepted what I said. I was spinning in my head, partly with sadness and partly with joy. I excused myself and drove home. I knew why I was telling the lie: to save time. It was a "white lie." I knew it would take an hour to explain why. The point came out the same. But, by God, I was "growing up." My brain was mending. I was in between total freedom and returning to "normal."

I called Mary Walsh immediately by phone. Bittersweet blessing.

Until then I had been able to drive, very carefully. I used the car only to drive to daily Mass at St. Cecilia's, and occasionally to Palmer's supermarket, where I would park as far away from everyone else as possible. Then, feeling so much better, I drove to my dentist's, in Springdale.

When I first visited Dr. Stein, Martin helped explain my problems. My speech was much improved, but it may have been the part of the head that was not able to communicate well.

"Put out your tongue" I had learned to respond to, but "Keep your mouth open" was difficult. "Put your tongue over on the right" left me baffled. "Up? Down? Spit?"

"The head is dead," I said.

But he found his own way of communicating Babel. He managed to make me feel almost cured. He was always praising my growth.

However, feeling daring, I started driving the car home, found a bit too much traffic, got nervous, and hit a parked car on the right. Panic! I had no idea what one did next. Son Paul, home for a break, rescued me from the total confusion. The insurance premium would go up, the car went off to the gas station's hospital, and I believed I would never drive again.

"It's like falling off a horse," the doctor said. "If you don't get right back on, you'll be too afraid."

"I thought my brain was getting better. But now—what is my chance of recovery of everything? I hate being half well."

Oh, shoot!

Like a prisoner, I felt that I had been moved from one jail to another. Maximum security was eased, but I wasn't free. I knew psychiatry well enough to know that if you have half a cup of water, you see what you expect to see. I felt half full.

My mother, Grace, used to tell me a verse her mother taught her:

> Patience is a virtue,
> Virtue is a grace
> And Grace is a little girl
> Who has a dirty face

Ginny and Alice were playing outside. I had done my piano lesson. I had spent fifteen minutes trying to remember how to work the typewriter. I had gone to the Weed Library to get some books.

"Help me find a book written about Patricia Neal, the actress, who had aphasia," I said. I, who was so darn' smart and in love with library skills, took a look at the filed cards and nearly cried out loud. Oh, pride! My mind was blank. I wandered into a corner, looking for a Kleenex. I saw a book of mine on the shelf. I picked it up and stared at it.

*House with a Hundred Gates, a Memoir.* I looked at Page 1. "My God! I don't know what it says."

The librarian brought me the book on Patricia Neal.

"What a beautiful woman she is! What strength!"

With Ginny I took out a book on nursery rhymes. I had a very drippy face.

Everybody knew about Patricia. She was on the commercial

for coffee. Her aneurysm and stroke were so much worse than mine; she had been pregnant in the middle of her illness. I was proud of her, and I keenly watched her. I saw her work as half full. I hoped she'd make it. But I kept hoping I could do better.

Oh, pride! I had been told that she had at some time walked into a house in England and felt her eyes return to normal. I wanted to read her husband's book. But when I brought it home, I could only browse through it. I couldn't really read it and make sense.

Only one book I could read, a book given me by Mary Walsh entitled *He and I*, a translation of the French *Lui et Moi*, by Gabrielle Bossis. That I could read, and understand. It was her memoir of talking with Jesus. With that I had no trouble.

My friends were so close to me that year! With Mary Walsh and Margaret Mary Cycon, who helped me to visit Cathy in her illness, I could go to Bridgeport and browse about in the bookstore of the Daughters of St. Paul. I looked at my most loved books, the new ones arriving, the oldest classics. I could not understand them. But I could get records of music, the monks of Weston, Sebastian Temple, the Franciscan, and the second part of Gabrielle's book. People are so kind to me. Back home I looked at *He and I*. Nearby was a book Mary Walsh had given me on St. Paul that I couldn't read.

"Do you remember your beloved St. Paul? His vision, his excitement, his wanting to get busy working?" said Jesus.

"You sent him back to his own town, and to his own work as a tentmaker."

"Well, you're not Paul. And you're not Gabrielle. You are a lucky nothing. Be glad, and grow up a little more."

"Grow up? I don't want to grow up. I'm safer as a child."

"The second chance is your purgatory. And you have so

much to relearn. The time before adolescence is harder, being a child. And try reading the French; it's better."

"I can't read French anymore. I can't even read the Bible in English."

"What I want done can be done."

With Ginny, I'd regularly be glued to "Sesame Street" and "The Electric Company." I was going to school from five to six every evening. Television, with its sounds and language, took my brain to a higher level. My intake of information needed to be speeded up. My output was fairly good. I could communicate what I wished to say. But memory was still locked in my brain.

Would I ever be able to teach again?

"Try it," said Ben. "Look up your notes on Buddha and see if you could present a lecture. Tell me what it was about."

I tried. Even I knew it wouldn't work.

Ben said, "You have pieces that you remember. You talk as if you were a poor translator, talking in another language. And there are large gaps in your brain. You can't go to school forever. But if you could get your friends from the college to help you, that would be better. Why not ask them?"

I needed "Sesame Street." And I needed lectures on a Ph.D. level. Enough intellectual stimulation could tie the strings in my brain cells. With Peggy Mooney I had gone up to the college for Mass at the chapel. People were glad to see me. But how can you ask someone to come and talk? There's no curriculum for teaching aphasics. Mr. Kidera, the president of the college, was very kind.

"You had just gotten tenure, and it's yours. You're still on the faculty. You're still on leave. Come over and see me whenever you can."

"Martin had bought me my cap and gown," I said. "I've never been able to wear it."

"Maybe at graduation this year? Meanwhile, why not sit in back at the lectures and see how it feels?"

I sat listening to my chairman teaching RS101. Then I thanked him and went home. I wasn't even at a freshman level.

Like any mother, I was praying for my children. A mother can at times see what should be done to heal or help a child. At other times, one can see nothing but a dark horror, with no hope ahead.

One night, I was naming each of the children.

"Pray for my child."

His voice was stern. "Whose child?"

I repeated my prayer.

"Whose child?"

"Your child, Lord! Not mine but Yours."

"They are all My children, including you. You are not a mother; you are a simple child."

I had never felt so free before. What a blessing when you finally realize you are not in charge at all.

"I pray for Your child. . . ."

"Then, I pray with you to the Father."

I am a member of the Third Order of St. Francis. I remembered that, as a fool for God, the saint did the nearest job to be done. He started fixing up an old, abandoned church. A servant doesn't wait to be told what jobs are around. Clare was in school, at Stamford Catholic High School. To raise money, the parents were going to have a large tag sale. My art was horrible, but I made posters and refreshed my memory of prices at antique stores and junk shops.

One can go to school for speech therapy for a while and then that's as far as you're going to go. Moneywise and timewise, Ben agreed I should quit. But aphasics need goals, need to sharpen their minds. For some it may help to look at their own attics and in their drawers, studying their usefulness to others. The mind, the fingers, the hands make exercise not a bore. One idea generates another.

"You're only half handicapped," someone said to me. "Stop every day and see what you can do half full."

I still wanted to write.

John Delaney, my kind editor, wrote me notes reminding me that I should write a book on aphasia. I felt touched, but kindness was not enough. John had invited me to lunch in New York, as if I were a writer. But inside myself I always said: I *used* to be a writer. Psychologically that is a horrible blow.

But John figured out my hang-up. "In the summer of '72 you agreed to write a book," he said, "and I gave you money as an advance."

"I yi yi!" I laughed. "Do you really want your money back?"

"No," said John. "I want you to write a book. Get going!"

It didn't seem possible. But one step at a time.

I had written down the story of St. Joseph. My language was misspelled. So I worked again at the dictionary. Then grammar? How do you handle that? There was no school for a half-ungrammared teacher. Or was there one?

Clare mentioned to me Sister Ledden, at school, a handicapped nun busy teaching and running the drama programs. She had time to hear me out. I had written it as a poem with refrains. Carefully, she helped me edit.

From one handicapped to another we asked what our physical problems were. After a summer of graduate work at Catholic University she had taken a Pullman sleeper on the way to

Montreal. She was in the upper bunk. The train collided with another. She saw real stars as her bunk bed went with her in it through the window of the train and crashed into the side of a mountain.

"With surgery, and X rays, it was clear that I could never walk again," she said walking around her office. "What does the Lord have to say: a miracle? I keep going back for checkups. The X rays say one thing; the facts say something else."

Swimming is fantastic exercise for aphasia, and up the street from our house was the Italian Center. Alice and Ginny and I would swim winter and summer. Ginny at two was a born swimmer, and apparently all Swedish women are great swimmers too. I was busy remembering how to co-ordinate. Cape Cod water was in my veins, but the right side constantly veered to the next lane. Oh, well! Summer came and I did better.

Jo Moran, come to visit, cheered me on.

Although we were separated by several states, visits with Jo and Bill were a marathon of fun and talking, with the total closeness of love. So often friendship between women is rewarding and charming. But to find married teams as friends is gorgeous. With the Mayglothlings and the Morans, what more could I ask for?

Except, they weren't swimmers, and they weren't teaching me humility. That I found in a handicapped person who had more gumption than I did. For years I had known Tom Meath, a paraplegic who lived down the street. He could not move. He could use his head; that was all. With polio at eleven he had ended up in an iron lung. With help and prayer he had graduated from college at Fairfield and gone to the University of Illinois, ending up with a master's in rehabilitation and patient counseling. With help, he had mobility to move in an electric wheelchair and worked, at Stamford's Health Department, with drug addicts. Later, when the Health Group was moved to another building, on the second floor with no elevator, Tom was again out of work. Determination? Partly, and partly God's grace. He, who could not feed himself, or move, who had to be carried and cleaned, who could not even drive away a fly buzzing, could help others. He could work on getting ramps to cross the streets and work for legislation necessary for others.

I came to admire him in the Italian Center. "Do you want to write a book about your life?"

"Yes, I've started it."

"I can't write. But I can help you, maybe. I have some savvy. May I read your notes?"

Strange groups God chooses. Margaret Mary Cycon, a school psychiatrist deeply involved in a rosary prayer meeting, was a close friend of Tom's, who really couldn't stand rosaries. However, Tom, a non-traditional Catholic, was deeply involved in helping with the counseling not only of other handicapped people but those emotionally handicapped by drugs and alcohol.

I, who was perhaps middle of the road religiously, could, as usual, help and be helped. From Tom I could take counsel on being handicapped. For him, I could get help for his writing. His book was never finished. It did not need to be done. Like all disabled people, he needed only to confess himself to himself. And for that he needed a guide.

I couldn't do that. But, for my birthday, I asked my brother for a wish. "You're overworked, much too busy, but would you as a great editor come to visit Tom Meath, and give him confidence and courage?" What a beautiful brother! Three times he came, reading Tom's manuscript. I sat back and listened. Watching an editor at work, I relearned part of the skill taught to me in the past.

The whole year of 1974 was a time of slow growing. In one way a new day always danced in, fresh, in voice—a present. With each moment there was the beauty even in pain, in confusion, in fear, in happiness. Is it aphasia that etches the brilliance even in the rain, the color of thirty-nine separate grays? Or is it having a child with one that lets one see growing life? With Ginny I would walk from the garden into the deep woods. Deep? Well, the walk was about thirty-five feet long, past one oak, five miniature apple trees, and two hemlocks. Or was it a forest, with the smell and sounds of a mysterious unknown? I would watch Ginny piggy-back on Martin.

"Poppy! Bring me around again!"

We were all growing. Cathy was strong enough to be with us for Ginny's birthday, and like any grandma I was astounded with joy: Jenny and Ginny celebrating a double birthday party. Violets covered the "forest" with messages of God's goodness.

And in another way the same new day was a reliving of the past, with a second chance. Many with strokes find that their memory operates on various levels of time. In 1973 I was singing songs of the twenties and thirties. In 1974 I was up to the fifties and sixties: I would see a grown child of mine and, flashed into my memory, I could see what I had been thinking and doing with that child in the past. It was scary but gorgeous. It was a confession of things I had not understood.

"Oh—if I had only understood!" I would say. "I'm sorry!"

"Whatever are you talking about?" said the son, over six feet tall. He had turned on the sprinkler outside.

"Because my brain sees you at another time, right here, when you were eight years old. You had been so awful around the house all day, exploding with all your brothers. I thought you were overwrought and you were going to use the hose to upset people. So I turned a light spray on you to cool your brain. I shouldn't have. I should have hugged you instead. I'm sorry. Forgive me."

Part of aphasia is the rewind of memory, *déjà vu*, sitting back and seeing it from a new view. Most of that whole year, I would make amends as the old and new parts of the brain began to mend.

But remember, this is Babel. I, going through different levels of my brain, made perfect sense *to me*. And yet, communicating in the present, I was not only kooky but also using language untranslated: "Oh, what a bore!" "Grow up!" and "Damn it to Hell!" A penance for all.

But time does not stand still.

Fulton went to Spain for his junior year at Georgetown. Clare went to school close to where Cathy was. Paul returned to Stamford Catholic High. And I was marking time, waiting till my sentence was over.

At the evening prayer meeting with Sister Ledden much kindness was given to me. One woman had told me of something I had said in a book.

"I have no memory of that."

So they told me what the book said. It was *House with a Hundred Gates*. I was fascinated, hearing my memoir.

"Hey, it wasn't bad for a book," I said laughing. "Was that really true?" Yes, it was true. But for at least a year after that I kept feeling it wasn't true: somebody else must have written it.

It was still very difficult for me to read at all, though at times I could read the Bible for five or ten minutes at a time.

I kept trying to finish that darn' word humility. But I couldn't.

What would I have done without Alice? Just as Mary Ball talked to me about getting out anger on the kitchen cabinets, so Alice, suffering with her bad foot, helped me talk out my frustration. We would end up rearranging furniture or rehanging paintings or singing "Ring-around-the-rosy-all-fall-down" with Ginny. Three children being nuts together. What fun being grandmas!

So often with stroke people, the past is clear, the present is clear, but the recent past is put in limbo for a while. Awareness occurred in 1973–74, but dates meant little to me until memory of the past was nearly filled, later.

At Advent I began sorting through the charming kindness people had given to me. Knowing my devotion to Mary and to Fatima, Mary Walsh and Al Riccio had even brought the international pilgrim statue of Our Lady of Fatima to our house. With the help of others, our house was often a place of worship and meditation. Father Peter came often, of course, and Father Tino, who had given me a plaque of St. Francis' Damian Cross. Here, too, Joey Lomangino, the blind man, came to lecture on Padre Pio and the rosary.

Strange, the forgotten time between present and past. As I went upstairs to our bedroom I realized the treasures, the blessings given to me. A woman I have never seen had loved my father's work. Ruth Graham had sent to me a large and beautiful modern painting of Our Lady of Guadalupe. Close to it was a Cybis sculpture of Mary with a blue jay. I sat on my bed with the prayer *Suscipe* in my hand.

I had seen, constantly, a relic of the true Cross tied to my bed. Father Peter had placed it with me in the hospital. It had been there in my playroom at home, that first year, before I could reach the second floor. It was still there with me when I finally looked at it and remembered.

"My God, how wonderful people are to me! How do I ever thank them?"

"Never enough," said Jesus. "You will never be able to remember all that they have done. You think so, but I give you this moment only, to see them clearly. Carry their kindness with you in your heart, and sing it at Christmas midnight Mass. But you will forget. You will be again a prophet of uselessness, feeling sorry for yourself, crying in Babel again."

"I will *never* forget to thank them," I said, seeing the faces of their charity.

"You and Peter! Right now I hold you in the center. But as a prophet you shall be let go again, sliding back and forth. Pride is on one side, loneliness and despair on the other. Only then will you understand how useless you are without Me. You will be alone in the boat with no keel. Without My word you know nothing. Cry Babel!"

Christmas was festal and holy. Exciting times were ahead. Cathy, so much better, had decided to have Ginny baptized. From across the river in New York State our family came for that special day, with Father Egan and Father Aquinas of Graymoor. In courtesy, Father Aquinas asked if, as a grandmother, I would read the epistle. I could not.

"Grow up," I said. "You know I can't read out loud."

Oh, what a bore!

## CHAPTER SEVEN

The brilliant winter, in snow, in ice, in wind. I exulted in life. Finches, blue jays, nasty starlings, and squirrels shook the acre with nervous, busy noises. Underneath the frozen and smooth surface of the stream ran a torrent, shaking, occasionally crackling through it, black water cascading up and over the shiny white. Opposites. In the air the trees sometimes screamed of death: an old tree lost a half-broken limb, unable to be coffined till spring. Under a nook on the south side, weed grass grew and the coleus damply whispered of spring.

When, once, real soft snow danced sweetly on our mittens, little Ginny and I made snowballs, and I taught her how to lie down carefully to make angel wings for others to see.

Isn't it funny how long it takes for children to get dressed to go out in the snow? By now I wasn't a little child any more. I could prove that I knew it took ten minutes to go out, fifteen minutes to play till we were frozen, and twenty-five more minutes to get undressed and changed, hanging up what must be dried. Cocoa, which I hate, had to be fixed for the child.

Ginny could sleep. But I was not ready for a nap. I wasn't a child any more. In my brain I was trying to know where I belonged. An ugly duckling? In a way, in half aphasia, I was. I certainly wasn't a swan. Mentally, it was better to see myself as a gawky early-teen-ager.

"What are your problems? What are your goals?" I would write down, "Let's be practical."

The first question was my health and my prognosis. Early in January, Dr. Ray examined me.

"I was awful angry at you last time," I said. "Maybe that gave me the spunk to try it. Tell me, how am I?"

"You're doing great. There are still changes growing. You've been working hard." He gave me the horrible test of things to be named. I passed perfectly.

"In the middle of a rehearsal in choir, I suddenly understood what nuts and bolts are. Things just suddenly click in the strangest places. *'Christe eleison*—nuts and bolts!'"

"Music. Not just the sounds and fun, but the awareness of wanting to work at something a bit hard," he mused. "I'll bet the Mass was a challenge. And that exercise pushed the brain."

"Doctor, my brain feels rusty, in need of oil. A word to be learned and remembered is like having a tack and a hammer and a picture. I don't co-ordinate well, so I keep dropping the tack or the hammer. But by the ninth try the picture is up and the word is grooved into my damn' head."

"Are you playing bridge?"

"When my son Mike comes over, we play five hundred or chess. Chess I can handle for up to half an hour. Parchesi I always win, though. It's ESP that does it."

"Are you still going to speech? I think there's not much more for you there. You can practice it by yourself, and talking with other people. Keep on trying to read. Slowly it may get better. Non-fiction is good. Novels are more difficult."

I felt so at ease with Dr. Ray that time. Having him around made me feel I would make it all the way back to life.

Then Dr. Ray said: "You know, I'm almost ready to retire. I'll see you for the last time in June. That's all."

"What else is new?" I said to myself.

I went back to the hotel in Manhattan and called John

Delaney. We had a wonderful talk. What a terrific editor, talking about my book on aphasia, encouraging me. And then, gently, John said that most probably he would be retiring within the year.

I hung up the phone. Panic hit me.

I walked out of the hotel and almost ran down Fifth Avenue, hardly looking at people. Then, seeing St. Pat's ahead, I walked into a luncheonette and sat in the back and drank three cups of coffee like a drunken bum. Then I got out a pad and pen and thought: "I've only got six months to get well."

Then I read it. And then, being truthful, I had to write down the fact that it wouldn't happen. And I wrote down the fact that everything was falling apart: My health. My so-called work. And—my family and my marriage. I crossed it all out. And then I wrote it again, and added: "Is everything falling apart?"

What do you do when a marriage is dying? The signs were showing through the desperation of our life together. I did not want to mention it even to myself, but in the beginning of that strange year I had to be truthful. We had been looking for a miracle, a reborn honeymoon with happiness ever after. We said little about it except when family problems surfaced.

Was it a happy family? No. Unreal tension, emotional strain.

Was it because of my illness? No. It was erupting before my illness. My being handicapped did not cause our problem. But it made it worse for all of us.

I felt horror coming closer to reality. I crumpled up the piece of paper and went over to St. Pat's.

"I wanted to have a good marriage. I wanted to be well. I wanted to write. I won't ever make any of it."

"Everything you have wanted will be taken away," said the Lord.

I sobbed. "I won't believe it."

Ruefully, He walked away.

I sat in the darkest pew until I calmed down. Then He was sitting with me.

"When you go home, look it up in Matthew. Remember what I said. I did not come to bring peace to the earth. It is not peace I have come to bring, but a sword. For I have come to set a man against his father, a daughter against her mother, a daughter-in-law against her mother-in-law."

"Why?"

"I told you before, in Luke. I have come to bring fire to the earth. Do you suppose that I come to bring peace on earth the way it is?"

He left. He is a strange God.

I walked over to The Lady Chapel and lit a candle. Here Martin and I had been married. Here were the memories of my father and mother. Every dream I ever had seemed to be gone.

I stood so quietly that a guy sliced the shoulder strap of my pocketbook and I grabbed it just in time. I could hardly carry it without the strap and walked out in a huff.

Yet, damn it, outside in the early twilight the world was *so* beautiful!

"Ashes, ashes, all fall down!"

Ginny was a charming singer, morning, noon, and night. She loved singing with gusto "Lord, have mercy!" three times for every response at the monastery in New Canaan. And most of all, anywhere, she sang "Jingle Bells"! Even Alice wanted to strangle her.

Much like her, I was working with every routine to the hilt. I exercised on the stationary bike. I did exercises on the floor, with Ginny and Geisty-dog. I studied my music. I spent half an hour a day working at the typewriter. The right hand and brain were so slow.

And I began studying anatomy with art. In meditation my body reminded me that I had no image of myself at all. Particularly, I had no real awareness of my whole body. Jenny and Ginny, my grandchildren, I could feel and see at once, because they were small enough to feel with my left hand. But I did not like my own right hand. It did not belong to me, except three of my fingers.

With Martin's help I bought some books and started studying with Frieda Shapiro, working with charcoal. As a student I was forced to use different muscles, to stand back from a typewriter or a pen and paper and actually physically "dance" what I wanted to sketch. I needed perspective in an outward way, not inward. My mind pictured me writing with just three fingers and my head. For several lessons I was very unhappy.

I asked Tom Meath to show me his art. It was good.

"How did you achieve your special task, learning to paint with your mouth?"

"I learned not as an exercise or a gimmick . . . but as a release from human ecstasy," said Tom. "Control is essential to all life. Perseverance, too. I had learned how to paint ceramics as a task. Color awareness was interesting. But to paint the unseen, to act out light, darkness, shading, and a dream is—?" He smiled. "My art is a way of being on stage!"

To be on stage, to be part of the theater, is a way of being holy and accepting life. "All the world's a stage"; so Shakespeare said, but the art of the stage is often lost to the handicapped. Great as television and movies may be, theater production is more human and alive. And the production may be very small and amateur as long as it is unbottled and alive. All great religions have liturgies that act out our beliefs. Who knows within ourselves our power to enact the grandeur of God?

One of the most meaningful moments came to me when I saw Rudolf Nureyev. And I was surely not a ballet fan.

It was Sue Agnes who invited me to see him in New York. The Agneses and the Armstrongs, friends for many years, were for the last few years entwined. Bob had had a stroke a few years before my aneurysm; and Bob and I both went to speech with Ben Cariri. Sue had helped Martin to learn the ropes of handling the handicapped's problems. Debonair Bob was a joy for me to talk with. And Sue, a busy woman, often went out of her way to take me out.

Sue and I had lunch with Martin at the Rainbow Room and then went to the matinee. I was a little nervous. Our seats were on the left, and I was sure I wouldn't really be able to see. (That's an aphasic being unsure of herself.) Going up and down the stairs frightened me. I was balking at the whole idea.

Then, suddenly, Nureyev was on stage.

Fear disappeared. Presence hit me with awe. It was like hearing Beethoven or Handel for the first time. It was like first seeing the Sistine Chapel. My God, what man is! I, who never really understood ballet at all, saw a new dimension of God, extolling Him in one human being.

On the way home to Stamford I remembered a song singing through my mind. The refrain was:

Dance, dance, wherever you may be,
I am the Lord of the dance, said He.
And I'll lead you on wherever you may be,
Yes, I'll lead you on in the dance, said He.

Some years ago I learned that the words were sung in the seventeenth century in what was to be the United States, and at Fordham I had found writings in the third century of Jesus as the dancer. As David danced before the ark, so Christians danced with intense awareness of body-mind hymning the universe.

Sue and I are not dancers, except in our own privacy. But as Tom painted and I sketched or sang, God filled us with mystery. To feel and respond is necessary for all handicapped people. To sit back and mope and refuse to be in the theater of life is blasphemy.

I was still trying to open my locked memory of knowledge. Dr. Philip O'Shea, close to his own ordination, had no time to teach me philosophy. He had visited me in 1974 with the early Greeks through Plotinus. He had returned once more and picked up with Kant, and for some reason with Bergson.

Can you picture the structure of my mind, with wide holes? More than anything, I wanted to remember theology. Timorously I called Father Nick Grieco.

"Who are theologians? What happened from Vatican I to today? I've looked in newspapers and magazines and I've never heard of these people."

Bless him! Once a week, I'd drive over to St. Maurice's Church and listen. With aphasia I didn't need a regular lecture. I needed to see the men's names written down, and to listen to the sounds and movements of a relaxed teacher *reminding* me.

"Remember Tillich? The Ground of Being? Ultimate Concern? I bet you didn't like Barth as much. Now, Rahner. . . ."

Here and there memories glimmered. Sometimes it was a famous joke that opened a large piece of memory. Or a memory of Pope John XXIII wanting to open the windows. But mostly it was hard work listening, relearning, memorizing names: Rahner, new hermeneutic, Bultmann. And slowly it melded.

I thank also Philip Scharper, who lent me his tapes on "Liberation Theology." For the first two and a half years, my brain could not register a talk without visual aids. But, because he was an old friend, I listened to his voice over and over and gradually I could carry a whole lecture in my mind. The brain was healing.

Inside myself I began to feel self-confidence returning. A close friend, Dominic Tranzillo, was interested in my poem about St. Joseph. To my amazement, he composed *The Song of Joseph* and conducted it at Holy Spirit Church, with a bass soloist and the choir. Part of me rejoiced. I was sure everything was growing back to normal.

And then, on a warm day, I drove over to Peggy Mooney's house for lunch. I was driving at twenty-five miles an hour, which was normal for me. I went past her street, where I should have turned.

My brain could not handle two big ideas at the same time. Ahead of me was a van turning in to another driveway. I should have braked. But I had never been taught how to brake since my illness. No one had taught me, because I used to slow down until inertia stopped the car. Seeing the van, my brain yelled DANGER. So I pushed both feet down hard. I hit the brake and the gas at the same time.

I totaled my car. Those in the van weren't really hurt. Blood was all over me. I turned out to need a few light stitches. The windshield was smashed. And my confidence was zilched. For the next year, that horrible car was in our garage, a reminder that I could not be safe doing anything. But reality can be different. Stifling the spirit can be a kind of suicide.

Martin was miserable, and so was I. We were both equal victims of circumstance. To try to live by the so-called rules was unreal. Martin was unable to run away from my beliefs, and unable to cope with his own with me.

To separate a marriage seems unkind, impolite, wrong—unfair to the unhappy family, unhappy to husband and wife. Yet, in fact, doctor, lawyer, and friends agree: We could not live together.

"You'll both get deeply sick. The two of you could get a heart attack, a nervous breakdown, or die."

We loved each other, but not in marriage. What one thinks is "correct" is so different from what is present. Both testaments cry out and the veil is split apart.

In many ways, I had hoped I would never have to mention this in the book. But I soon realized it was necessary to help others. We were both victims, and we both cared for each other. Martin was kind, honest, trustworthy, full of faith, hope, and charity. I hope the same was true of me. But the marriage had died.

The viburnum smelled overwhelming at the front door. The lilacs and the irises were joyful. Ginny was picking dandelions, her hands stained with warm greenness.

"Jingle bells, jingle bells! Jingle all the way!"

She ran to Alice, who had her foot in a cast, and filled her lap with the blossoms.

Friends were kind, as usual. With Carol Dugan, I'd spend a day with my gifted godson, Kerry, and talk about biofeedback and mind control, and the possibility that I might someday go back to work. A new friend had been bringing me to the Third Order of St. Francis, in Villa Maria.

"What are your summer plans?" people would say.

"I don't know," I'd say.

And Ginny, forgetting "Jingle Bells" at last, smiled and said, "Dance with me. I like it. 'Ashes, Ashes. . . .'"

For almost three years I had seen the trauma of my illness as a separate entity. Fix that, and everything else would vanish. Look in the right book, follow the right guides. Sounds simple, but it's not.

Marital problems, particularly of seeing the world differently, don't disappear with a physical problem. A hiatus of illness does not change the game of marriage. In many books the rules are clear: if you are good and kind, and trying well, and pay, everything will work out.

The separation of a marriage is a horrible dance.

Each grown child was living through the thunderstorms of disintegration, with anger and pain and confusion exploding one against another. To each, to Paul, Clare, Caedmon, Fulton, Cathy, Mike, and Marty, I give thanks for caring. My beloved daughter-in-law, Kathleen, would come help me with the most important need, the ability to cry out love. Alice, who had real problems with her foot and so was unable to help care for Ginny, brought the ability to pray. Then, in the middle of other problems, Clare needed surgery. And Helen Mayglothling was right at my fingertips, driving me back and forth to New York. The nightmare of this year slowly changed the picture. Cathy was healed enough to be a full-time mother. The large house was empty except for me and Paul and little old Geisty.

Real friends are part of our opposites, bonded with love. If we're hungry, they feed us. Bud Mayglothling is a darn' good chef. If we're lonely, they comfort us. Helen was always around, going to the pool, driving me, calling me. And when we need guidance, they find a happy way.

Bud, however, got angry at me. "You're not writing. Every time you wrote a book, you would bring it over to my house. Helen would collate copies and we'd both tell you how great you are, *because you are*. And now you aren't writing."

"I can't! I used to. But it's over. I can't."

"Yes you can. You will. But, damn it, you might give up. And I can't stand that!"

Boy, I loved Bud.

Jo and Bill Moran are the same kind of people. Are all great friends also chefs? Bill cooked steaks, told the best jokes, and said I was no longer sick but well. And I should get back to work. Jo, a terrific language teacher, talked about novels, college problems, and changes in the Catholic Church.

But I still didn't believe in myself.

By chance? It is something I do not believe exists. The seeds of our life are sown at the correct time, growing, and harvested as time occurs.

"What will you do with yourself, or your life?" some asked.

At least now I could read, slowly. And I had found my favorite books, books taught to be by Father Marius McAuliffe, o.f.m. Twenty years ago, when he was at Our Lady of Perpetual Help in New Canaan, he had directed me. One book more than others: Caussade, *Abandonment To Divine Providence*. Slowly I reread it and partly understood.

"I don't know what will happen. But my job is to see, and rejoice, and do what is to be done. The pachysandra needs pruning. And the weeds are overtaking the flowers."

Not by chance, I needed guidance psychologically and spiritually. Through Helena and Joe Rich and music I came to know Father Al Sienkiewicz, pastor of Holy Spirit Church. Father Al's psychological studies, including aphasia and the problems of speech, gave me deeply needed confidence as he gently pushed me to express words. Friend chauffeurs made my weekly conferences with him possible.

Father Al was, among other things, instilling confidence in me to talk with others. I would start to say a word I wanted to use and was unable to see the word in my mind, so I'd stumble, looking for a simpler word.

"Say it, whether it makes sense or not. I want to hear it."

Pride scared me, but I would say it. It sounded a bit like it.

"Try it again. Do you think it might have been . . ."

No pride, just hesitation, quietly spitting it out. Tears would fill my eyes.

"Missassessom." Or "Lit-lit-chush." Kindly, he corrected them: mysticism, liturgy, humility.

And along the way, he healed much of my misery, telling me I was good. Oh, how much we handicapped need to be told we are good! Good at anything! I suppose some of us can, at times, become overriding and nasty. But, to heal, we must be filled with love, and then we can be shown our unloveliness and we can work with our problems.

Not by chance, Father Roderick Brennon, c.o.f.m., director of our Third Order of Franciscan Minors group, called me for help. I could not help him, but I found Peggy Mooney to solve Father's problem. And then I told Father of the marriage being splintered. Father Roderick stopped by my home to sit with me, listen to my unsolved problems, and soothe me. Not by chance, but by providence, I needed help from that priest right at that moment. What fun it is to see the mysterious movings of God! I feel so sorry for those who see a burning bush and do not notice it.

Not by chance, Margaret Harris suddenly called me. We were both friends of Father John de Marchi, i.m.c. Margaret, a writer and a convert, had given her large house to the Convent of St. Brigitta's, in Tokeneke. She had offered it first to the Consolata missionaries, but it was better suited as a hospice and retreat. Margaret picked me up.

"You should meet Sister Louise," she said. "A *young* nun."

And young she is, eighty-five years old. Eleven years before she became a nun at last, a gal with worldly savvy, having helped and raised her own grandchildren, widowed, she had finally found a new life in the Lord. We belonged together as friends. I had been hoping to go back to Regina Laudis but did not know how to do it. But now with joy I knew it was time for me to rest on retreat at Vikingsburg.

"What are you coming for? To rest? To be opened? And direction?"

"Yes. Whatever comes. Wouldn't it be great if the Lord would set a course and tell me exactly what my life is for?"

Her Texas drawl was charming. "You know that won't happen. He has such peculiar ways. But the food is good and the guests are nice and I love you."

So it was that I sat in the shade on the crag of the tiny hill meditating on the beauty of the seaweed. Here the fresh-water river and the bay of the sea meet. The heavy, life-and-death stink of low tide delighted my soul. It was as close to my memories of Cape Cod as I could get.

Closing my eyes, I reflected on my body, then, moving on to another meditation level, I let go and felt safe. Jesus was sitting with me.

"You have loved St. Francis so much! His prodigal love for Me—Francis, the fool's herald."

I saw Francis dancing, singing, with animals and birds, the morning light of the sun, the mystery of water so close to his awareness. And his childlike delight—as in starting the crèche idea.

"You do love him so much," said He again, "because you try to be like him, saying of Me: 'My God and my all.' You have done the best you can, trying to understand him. You have thought about the seraphim who gave Francis the stigmata, the wounds of My Heart. But you have not really seen the human paradox. Look at him. He was miserable—not by pain but something worse. Feel what Francis felt."

The rush of the wind blew over the rocks below. Francis made it clear.

"Oh, my God! Francis, who wanted to be humble, was put on display. He could not hide Your wounds. I *never* thought how awful that was. The pain, the rapture of sweetness sharing with You—that was all right. But . . . to be festooned so he could not seem humble! Why not do it silently, unnoticed? That's what he wanted. When You went to Golgotha nobody knew it but Mary. But . . . for Francis that was the worst cross, wasn't it?"

"Yes," said Jesus.

I had not understood what the last twist of horror was: the awareness of being known to all, cultivated as a famous saint on display. Like Mary, the humble servant who had to be known to others.

"Mary, and Francis, had to lose their last piece of pride."

The tide was turning.

"You see that," He said, standing. "But you still have not seen it all. Paradox is what you have to learn. It will take you time to see. Look now at Anthony."

I saw the son of Portugal who wanted to be a missionary and ended up in Italy instead. He accepted that, and wanted to be a scullery man in the Franciscan monastery. He ended up as a theologian. Parable of paradox; the least becomes the highest. Then I saw Anthony giving a homily and seeing Jesus as a child sitting on Anthony's arm.

"Not that, Lord!" I cried.

"Yes," He said. "Stately Anthony, imbued with Me as the Savior, the Cross, the Resurrection? Yes? But for him to accept Me as a child. Other people in the Church could see Me on Anthony's arm, see Me as a sweet little child."

"Poor Anthony! Why?"

He chuckled. "You think I mixed them up? That I should have given Francis the vision of Me as a child? And Anthony the stigmata? Oh, child, you do not *yet* understand. The opposites are always true."

"And people miss the point too," I said. "I hate those prayers for St. Anthony to find lost things, or asking for favors to be done. He was a great theologian, a great teacher, not a sticky-sweet man. It's like the Infant of Prague, so dainty. My mother loved those statues, with clothes to change. I couldn't stand them. What were You really like as a child?"

"The opposite. You know I was a good Jewish boy."

"You don't fit with our ideas. You are not *good* in our way of seeing what we *think* is good."

"True. But if you're open to Me I break through to you. The glass breaks so there is room for Me to take over. What you people least expect—that is the Trinity, loud and clear, upsetting so-called reality. Wait. You'll see."

The trouble was that in no way could I see anything that made much sense. And during it all, I began to realize that some people thought I had an obsession, an obsession with God. I talked about God as though He was real. And slowly I began to understand that few really do.

I was always singing to God. I was watching life and reacting to God. I was feeling life with God. And when I worked I would look up from time to time and notice the weather, or a bird, or the color of something, and share it with Him.

"For God's sake, can't you ever think of something else? Religion is fine, and it has its own place. But really—you're sick."

I don't talk about it constantly. But I sort of breathe God, and I think of Him always. If you believe in your creed, what else is there? Then everything else fits together.

But, for safety's sake, I learned to be a bit more quiet. I realized I was a freak, enjoying the presence of the living God.

"She's on a kick, you know. She's always going to church."

My hunger for God was everywhere. I needed to be filled daily in the Eucharist, the moment when eternity and time are fused. Many others go to daily Mass. Isn't that normal?

"It's a psychological problem, filling their ego. She's always talking to priests. She ought to be a priest."

Oh, no.

I walked my way through the woods and up the steep gravel to the monastery. I ordered myself to stop talking or singing so much when others were around. If nothing else, I could end up in a nuthouse.

Tired, breathing heavily, I rested next to a parked car. It was a few minutes before Mass time. I looked at the nearly frozen asters.

"They're beautiful," He said.

I looked at Him and closed my eyes. "Go away."

"So they think you're crazy! Who cares? Look at Me."

Even with my eyes closed I saw Him. I opened my eyes.

"Walk with Me so you won't be late."

He seemed to be about thirty years old this time.

He took my left hand. "Come on."

He was wearing, for some reason, a Franciscan robe, but His was dark, dark gray. I was taller than He was. And I felt as though I was falling apart.

Then He left and I stared at my hand. *Oh, God, I'm crazy.*

"Hi!" An acquaintance was on her way to Mass too. Then she said: "You look upset. What's the matter? Oh, no. You look very happy. I guess I was wrong."

"I don't know. But we're almost late."

At the Consecration, one kneels, but soon after, in the Byzantine Rite, one stands again. I was shaking.

"What more can I do?" He said to me. "Here is My Body. Here is My Blood. Do you believe in Me?"

In the line to receive, I kept looking at people around me. At Brother X, and Brother Augustine. They didn't seem to see anything unusual. I shook.

"Will you not eat of Me? I am spilling My own love, and you do not wish Me? Would you step back again? Will you bow and run away? Run to Me. Drink with Me. Soul to soul."

The priest usually calls us there by name, and waits for us to accept.

"Amen." What else could I say?

One priest I knew well nodded at me afterward. Father Philip O'Shea and others in the Third Order were having donuts. "You have a problem," said Father Philip.

"I have."

"I know. And I'm not the one to help you."

I started to look at the chapel. I looked at my hand. "I don't know."

"Yes, you do." Father Philip gave me a donut and a cup of coffee. "Have a safe walk home. I'll think of you."

I needed so much help. Money, thanks to Martin, was not a problem. But I needed time to grow, time to feel needed, time to be taught, and time to see my faults.

One thing I needed desperately I found again. AlAnon. Alcohol was not Martin's problem at all. In no way was that why I was returning to AlAnon. As I had explained in another book, alcohol was a disease from my mother's family line, cured, by God, in AA. Bill, the famous founder, and his wife, who started AlAnon, taught my father and me the lessons to be learned. The non-drinker is the real problem in every family, too darn' perfect to be useful to God. The parable of the Prodigal Son is for AA. But the elder son in that parable was a show-off, a bore, with love buried in so-called perfection. The AlAnon message says, Let go and let God run you. One day at a time! I called and asked for help at the handsome Presbyterian "Fish" church in Stamford. It's the cheapest and best therapy available.

At Thanksgiving, Father Peter Mongiano, I.M.C., my frequent visitor in the hospital, returned as usual, *Deo gratias.* With Mass in our living room we gave thanks for the year. Talking with him later I said, "It was a lousy year. It was also a good year. I don't know whether anything belongs. Help me to know."

"Just be still. He will tell us each when the time is right for something to be done. That's all. Not a moment before. 'This is the day the Lord has made. . . .'"

"'Let us rejoice and be glad in it!'"

As was our usual habit, we played records and sang along with them.

In trying to write, I found that part of my unconscious level was ready to open. In explaining my memory of the aneurysm, I found myself writing out the pain, the fear, the fury, the rage back in 1972. With nobody around, I acted it out, using every strength of my adrenalin. Then I fell asleep, and worked some more. Excitement, a volcano, bottled-up emotions came out in spasms. It was as if pus had to be acted out, spat out as if in convulsions. It was as if my body needed to act out everything: my nose had a tainted, foul smell, the stench of vomit. My mouth was blackish, like warm, insipid water after taking nasty pills. And I wanted to break everything. A woman on a rampage.

Oh, boy! What fun! What glorious fun! I was on an awfully high kick of psychological awareness. I had finally broken open the barrier of my memory.

I called Dr. Casey at St. Joseph's Hospital. Even over the

phone he heard the change in my voice. When I came to visit him he could see the change: I was standing, moving differently, much like my old, normal self. We talked about many things. Then he said: "Would it interest you to come to a stroke symposium next month?"

"I know nothing about stroke people. I haven't had a stroke."

He nodded. "But you would be interested in the work at the Easter Seal Center, with speech pathologists and so on. Some doctors are talking about aneurysms and aphasia. I think you ought to come."

"I will." And went back to writing.

With Christmas over, Chris Golightly drove me up to Regina Laudis for a New Year's retreat. I was reading Thomas Martin's *Wisdom of the Desert,* resting in almost silence in St. Gregory's House. *What will the new year bring?* I asked. *Something special!*

Early after the Latin Mass, December 31, 1975, I walked outside and suddenly started to shout. "Oh, my God. I can see three dimensions in my eyes!"

I ran to the trees, touching them. I ran to the snow, giddy, yelling. A priest walked by and I laughed.

"Look at them!"

"Yes, ma'am." Oh, well! One doesn't usually make so much noise. I stamped out to the steps to the eating room. Mother Assumption was getting things ready for breakfast.

"I can see three dimensions."

"You're what, April?"

"For the last three years everything in my eye has been only two-dimensional. Flat, like a postcard. But now, see! The Lord has let me see that. Look at that tree. Oh, look at that bottle of honey."

"God is good."

"But you don't really know what that looks like when it has been taken away. It was useful, because I could guess how far things were away from me. But now it's *real!*"

My boots dripping, I hurried outside again. I nuzzled the tree with ice and snow. I could see there were some tiny dead branches in the living tree. It was like being healed of blindness.

God! May I never again forget little things we take for granted.

I told Mother Placid.

"Did it come back like Pat Neal, the actress?" she asked. "Or is there still part of the eye that won't work on the right side?"

"Who cares? Of course, I can't see *everything*. Part of both eyes is lost. But oh, if you could see what I can see now. Look at the rail. Look at your hands! Look at my hands! Look at my feet. Look at where they wrote this note: +Pax. It stands out in front of the wall. It's just a tiny piece of paper with a tack, but it is bigger than the wall behind it."

I stared at my arms. "By God, the arm on my right side looks real. Maybe I will begin to believe I exist all the way."

"You are real."

"But I seldom see that right arm. And I've never yet seen all five fingers on my right side at the same time. I can see four, but one or another is missing. See, I still have to guess what the other finger is doing." I felt sad again for a minute. Then I rejoiced again. I noticed my coat and saw it as three-dimensional and was fascinated.

"Whatever the new year brings, may I take nothing for granted!"

## CHAPTER EIGHT

The year 1976 was a year of growing, in the Easter Seal Center and at Sacred Heart University. I needed help, discipline, and confidence to get back into normal life.

Early in January, Peg Mooney and I went over to Mass at Sacred Heart University again. The chapel, a bit run down, is not unusual, in need of refurbishing. But the presence of that chapel is warm and holy. And it was the center of almost twelve years of my life. I wanted to be there.

"I wonder," said Peg, always looking at the practical side. "You do have tenure, teaching there, don't you? You really love teaching. But you don't have to."

At that time I couldn't really explain it totally. But I knew that even if I could not teach, I wanted to be part of Sacred Heart. Bishop Walter Curtis, of Bridgeport, had a dream of the first Catholic laymen's college for commuters. It was dangerous, difficult, and exciting, and many like me were drawn by his vision, proud to be part of fulfilling it. To translate Cardinal Newman's idea of a university to the middle class, with no dorms, meant students who study, drive home, and go to work. Growing pains rampaged. The Catholics in Bridgeport had just built a new high school. Some were dismayed and really angry when the bishop turned it into a college. Many thought it was unreal, a waste of time, a second-class idea that would not jell, falling apart quickly. It did not. Then, why?

In many ways the whole meaning of the Sacred Heart was a

parable to me. What things are, and what they appear to be, are always spiraling opposites.

"There's a feeling of peace in that chapel," said Peggy, noting the ceiling needed paint. "What peace!"

The chaplain at that time was John Giuliani, a thin, artistic soul influenced personally by Thomas Merton. In the tall, skinny windows, statues by Ilsa Niswonger gave the simplicity of earth met with the silent presence of eternity. The haunting music of Sister Patsy Deignan's guitar, much of it composed by herself, completely harmonized the liturgy of the epistles and the gospel. I had known her when she was a student in some of my classes in the past.

At lunch, I reminisced with the first chaplain, Martin McDermott. He's the exact opposite of Father John, a tall, robust man (for years he and I were always going on a diet), but another beautiful man, so imbued with the Sacred Heart! More than anything, I remember his quoting Elizabeth Browning on the unnoticed awareness of God while others sit and eat blackberries.

"You really believe you belong at Sacred Heart, don't you?"

I hadn't enough rational words to explain why. But part of it had to do with the very words "Sacred Heart." As a grown convert of the Church I had not liked the name or pictures of it. They really horrified me. I saw them as sticky-gooey, unmasculine, red hearts pumping away. I had read about it carefully, studied it theologically, and nodded politely. Then, some years ago, when I lived next to St. Ignatius' Church in Manhattan, the pastor, Robert Gannon, s.j., introduced me to the real understanding of the Sacred Heart. There was a special religious affair climaxing a novena. The church was filled to capacity. Gannon kept finding more places for people at side altars.

"April, stand right there. Don't fall. You're tall. Yes!" He pushed me up against the Sacred Heart. "If you have to, hold on!"

I guess, from that long hour, I began to understand. The language of piety is at times awful. But the translation of the living blood of God is truthful. *Sacred?* In English the word has become almost forgotten, a sound, rather than the silent meaning. The *Heart* is too much confused with medical problems to remember that Jesus is living still, with a real body, not in fantasy but in real humanity. That's scary to those who really think about it. Too often, Catholics use the words like rote, droning away, and don't know enough to be afraid, let alone awed.

To try to explain that, and try to add the idea of the university, or wondering if I could go back to teaching there, was difficult.

"I know I'm not ready to teach. But maybe sometime I'll make it. Having a goal is a good idea."

"You'll make it, then," said Peggy.

Calmly I went to the stroke symposium Dr. Casey had suggested to me. Halfway through the first session, I heard of the work at the Easter Seal Center in Stamford, of how therapy was explained to the patients. When I pictured the work done in occupational therapy I almost felt like screaming, like yelling, like bursting out in tears, like crying with joy. Without a word, I thought I would explode.

For three and a half lousy years I had had to find my own method of teaching myself. At the Easter Seal Center the teachers help the patient to get back to normal life: getting dressed, learning personal hygiene from hair to toes, being taught how to cook and how to pick short cuts to handle difficult problems.

When I heard this I had to run outside and let out the noises shaking me. *Oh, God, why did I have to work so hard without help?* Then, laughing, I ran back in to hear more.

On a break I found Dr. Casey. "How come I didn't know about it? Can I get into that place? How, tell me, how?"

It was really simple. Get an appointment, and let them explain it to me. Some have to pay, although it is not terribly expensive. Very often, insurance and Social Security disability policies may cover the cost. What I needed was an examination from my own doctor.

"Why do you want to go?" asked Dr. Nagle. "What can they do for you after all this time? Isn't it possible that you don't need it?"

Many doctors are not aware of facilities from our own government. Many don't have the time to look in on all the help available; and I don't blame them. The responsibility belongs to the laymen to do their part. And the middle class in this country has a strange disease of false pride, sick pride that believes only the poor go to government agencies. Way back, Martin had decided that it was best for me to be helped privately. It was more genteel. Was it part political view as a conservative, not liking public help? I really don't know all the angles, and I do know many good conservative families who agreed with Martin. All I did know was that I wanted help. It would take time, and red tape. But I believed that at last I could get there.

While waiting, I realized I had not been reading the newspaper well, one of my exercises. It was my father's birthday, and thinking of him and his deep interest in the Catholic press, I picked up the Stamford *Advocate* and forced myself to read it. In Letters to the Editor, Joan Fitzpatrick explained that the UP reported a hearing coming on the FCC banning religious services on the radio. She asked people to write and support the need of the ill, the infirm, and the homebound. The air waves, she said, must be free for those who live on faith.

Without services on the radio, I would have been miserable in the first months of my illness. Immediately, I wrote a letter to Washington. And then, to thank the writer, I called up Mrs. Fitzpatrick. Not by chance, we found much in common. Then, suddenly, in her excitement over the phone, she found herself unable to talk, as though her brain had lost the pattern.

"Do you have aphasia?" I asked. I explained what it was.

"I never heard of that. But I had a car accident eleven years ago. I wonder if that might be part of it. I was almost kooky with it for a long time, and I still ramble, talking. Too many ideas in my mind at the same time and—"

"We've got to get to know each other. What were you doing when you got sick?"

"Bill Fitzpatrick and I were pioneering a dream, a hotel for the elderly on limited incomes. We bought an eighty-eight-unit hotel to house, feed, entertain, and love. It's a crazy word for other people, but Bill and I mean real love, love for God. Well, anyway, we bought the hotel and in the middle of that my car accident confused the problem. Poor Bill!"

Many aphasics are overachievers, perfectionists, excited with life before having a stroke. They have been hard workers, motivated to strengthen all their skills. "And it's interesting, not all but quite a few with aphasia are deeply religious people," I mused. Anyway, Joan got some books on aphasia out of the library, and I studied all about Park Manor. The hotel, in the main part of Stamford, surely wasn't swanky, but I loved the people and the Fitzpatricks' dream. Immediately, I could see how I could help them and help myself. I became the Bingo lady on Wednesdays. One of my real aphasia problems was putting together in my brain numbers said out loud to me, and understanding them. Looking at numbers, I know what they are. Repeating them out loud, like reading out loud, uses an entirely different mechanism in the brain.

"I'll call the numbers loud and clear," I said to the players. "You know, I'm a good actress and I'll use all kinds of characters. But you have a job. You have to notice when I make a mistake."

"You're kidding!" a sweet old lady said. "You're not perfect? I never heard anyone pretend they're not really perfect."

I called Bingo with the voices of Ireland, of Brooklyn, of Long Guyland, of Atlanta, and Mrs. McGillicuddy's crazy puppet. Nobody could get bored with that. And along the way, by gosh, I'd see B12 and say out loud B21 and my friends would pounce on me. I was working hard mending my brain. The non-perfect helped the non-perfect and had a ball for weeks with Bingo.

How much I could learn from the elderly! Were they lonely? Not as much so as I. I needed to be useful. I needed to be taught. The wisdom of the old, their proverbs, their knowledge of work and of the past, are distilled in their words. Sadly, few have the time to listen.

I love them all at Park Manor, but most of all I loved Jacob Cohen. He looked a lot like my father, who had no Jewish blood in his line all the way back to A.D. 1066—all English. But, like Oursler, Cohen was excited with life, in love with God, well read, and shining with wit and dry humor that hit you like a dueling mark. *Touché!*

I had been playing records for others, who wanted to sing some modern religious songs. Cohen had sat and watched. When they left, he let me know that he knew the Torah, the Talmud, and the New Testament. "What do you think of Job? Your Jesus quoted it and used it. Why?"

To get into that discussion thrilled me. The next time, I brought my Torah. "Will you get yours?" I asked.

"No. I do not need it. My eyes are almost useless, just enough to take a walk outside. The other day in my room I believed for a moment I had really gotten my vision back. I watched myself reading the Torah out loud and thought I had a miracle. But it was a mirage. I closed my eyes and still could see myself reading it out loud."

We talked about Scripture, and we talked about life before I was born, his childhood in Brooklyn learning how to make dresses. From the cramped home, that family made beautiful clothes sold at Lord and Taylor's in Manhattan. In books and movies I had an idea of what life was like then, but luckily I now had a grandpa to share it with me. His dignity and charm gave me confidence and love.

The Fitzpatricks themselves helped me too. Joan and I would talk in the midst of confusion in a normal hotel. Having studied aphasia, Joan and Bill found it easier looking back on her illness when both lawyers and doctors believed there was nothing wrong with her. She had, for example, bought tons of clothes for her children, and gotten angry over small things with the family.

"Sometimes we thought she was pretending," said Bill. "I loved her, but she kept asking me to do things that weren't necessary. She was nasty and bossy. And at the same time she seemed to pretend not to know how to talk clearly, saying she couldn't remember what she was talking about."

"One of my children still believes there is nothing wrong with me, that I'm only pretending," I said. "Do you know what Babel is?"

So few Catholics know the Old Testament, or even the New, for that matter—but Mr. Cohen knew it. Though not a rabbi, he knew that Babel had a connotation of Babylon, where men forgot God's covenant. Babel was, of course, a symbol of everything of pride and of all evil. The Hebrew word *balal* was a pun, for *balal* meant literally "confound." In literal language we might be able to say: "God confounded our speech, confound it!" or "God confounded our speech, and we're stuck with it, damn it!"

Mr. Cohen shook his head. "We're always trying to be show-offs, running the world instead of letting Him run us. We can get to know ourselves only when we first get to know Him."

"To translate Babel, I think, is part of why I'm here," I said.

"You're a theologian. I ask you a question: Do you think there should be women priests?"

"No! Not me. I can't prove it. But I know it's wrong."

"There are women rabbis."

"Women's Lib is necessary for some people, I guess. I was taught to be a person, not a man or a woman, but just a person. In the Talmud we know wonderful judges—people—and some were also women. The fear of the Lord can rest on many prophets and many teachers, and they are open to the Lord and He uses them." It was time for me to call Bingo, and I gave him a kiss.

"Wait," said Cohen. "Aaron was a priest. His sister Miriam was a prophetess. I ask you: If you believe Jesus makes priests to offer bread and wine, is that meant only for men? *Why?*"

"It's time for Bingo!" I smiled.

"That's a job. But your real job is to get back to work! You are a theologian!"

"Not me," I said. But my mind was filled with excitement. I felt alive.

Within the next few days at home, some people, not by chance, called. "April, what do you think of the charismatic group?"

In one way, I remembered all about it. In another way, I had to be retaught the word. Strangely, it was usually those who were against something who were interested in asking me.

So-called traditional Catholics were upset. They did not know their Testament well, and they had not been taught much about the Holy Spirit, but they were afraid of heretics, and they were particularly afraid of defaming the Eucharist.

I thought. I decided I was not at all a theologian, but I was capable of finding out what was bothering my so-called traditionalists. I found a more modern gal and asked for a ride to a charismatic meeting.

My rusty brain was rehearing, rewatching, rethinking. Whatever your work used to be before injury, the same method is still there. My job was religion. Someone else's could be banking, or law, or being a stewardess or a mason. Physical movement is only part of our life. Mental excitement, for the injured, stirs us, a half memory of unwritten knowledge.

I went to the meeting. On the way into the meeting there were two vessels to place hosts for the Mass: one for Catholics, the other for non-Catholics. Pewter was for Catholics, gold for others.

"Why?" I asked.

"Gold will not be consecrated. We use pewter to consecrate, because so many are coming."

The priest was refreshing my memory of my dissertation. I found my notes from graduate school, four tomes full, and my head hurt physically. Just as Dr. Ray had said: Work hard mentally to get back your faculties.

The so-called modern Catholics asked why I didn't join this larger prayer meeting. And at the same time they asked me: "For goodness' sake, why do you go to the evening First Friday Mass? They're back in the old ages. And can you imagine having Benediction and a Holy Hour right after Mass? Mass is more important, but most of them are glad after Mass with all their devotions!"

I agreed in many ways. To honor the Blessed Sacrament was

to many more real than the whole Mass. To me it was like having a big cake and eating it all, and then holding up another cake that you can't eat.

"It's too rich for me," I said to a traditionalist.

Her anger erupted. "I want things back where they used to be. The Church is often causing problems. I bet some heretics will try to have women priests. Would you?"

"No."

"April, would you come to see the mystic on Long Island? We go by buses. She says the modern Church is taken over by the devil himself."

"I wouldn't go to see her. What I've read in a magazine makes me feel she's wrong. But why run around on merry-go-rounds, starting fights? Jesus *is*, in the Gospel, in the Mass, in us."

"I bet you're a women's libber," she said.

I bit my tongue. I had been sitting back feeling sorry for myself without pushing hard enough. A banker and a mason both remember what they were taught in school. They listen to what new teachers say. But, knowing unwritten knowledge, they respond with a wiser view. To push on into life, I would have to work hard, learn words, and attempt to communicate.

Over coffee at Park Manor, Bill and Joan were involved in elder citizens, the government, HEW, and politics.

"It's a rat race!" said Joan. "I should quit. But I won't, God knows why. I've been writing letters till I'm blue in the face. When I let some people left homeless after a fire come into our hotel, people thought I was wrong. If you do something kind, people look for motives. If you talk about the Gospel and take it literally, they think you're crazy."

"Hooray! You get angry at the Lord. You're alive. And you mean business when you talk to Him. If you're called 'Kooky,' let it be!"

She laughed. "Why were you talking about jigsaw-puzzle pieces?"

"I see it that way," I said. "It's like a huge puzzle. And you have some of the pieces. And I have some, stuck in my pockets, and some dropped on the floor. If we join ourselves, some of the pieces fit. And though we can't see the drawing of the picture, which is lost, and we're not sure what it looks like, we just have to see what's around."

Mr. Cohen came in from a walk.

"I've been reading your Gospel. You're good at parables. But tell me more about your Jesus. You've never tried to convert me, thank God. And you do believe our Lord made me in the covenant. But if you believe in Jesus, and you do, tell me, are you scared?"

I looked at Mr. Cohen. His age was bending his head. I usually kneeled to talk with him, and then he would insist that we must find chairs and sit together. But this time he stood, and I sat on the floor.

"When you talk about Jesus you are often radiant, joyful. You believe. But there is something bothering you. Talk to me. Do Catholics really talk to the Lord when they are nervous? Do they believe they can talk to Him?"

"Many don't really. They are too scared. They don't really believe all the way. They think it's not polite. They believe they are baptized, so they believe Jesus Christ is within each one. But they—"

"But they think it too simple to be true?"

I burst out laughing. "God loves you!" I stood up and kissed him.

"Oh, how awful!" He winked. "Yet I wonder why you are nervous. What do you think Jesus looked like?"

Memory brought back to my mind the Holy Shroud, the strange piece of cloth in Turin supposed to be the burying gar-

ment. I promised to show him a book on the Shroud with all
the data and a picture of what some believe was His face.

March, the time of in-between, the blue newness of squill
and snowdrops, the black and dirty ice and snow. My baptism
day is always close to a blizzard. How much like Holy Mary's
Day, March 25, the strange winter-summer time, the gusts'
fiery strength subdued by warm stillness.

One routine in my life was to catch Poltergeist and put him
in the house so I could walk to the monastery. Geisty wanted
to take care of me, of course. But larger dogs could start a
deathly fight. Once I lured Geisty in with goodies, I could
walk, briskly as the doctor taught me. Deep breathing, singing
loudly, strengthened the muscles of the heart. It was exciting,
watching out for branches, squishing in thawed springiness,
and the wind, sometimes turning me sideways, blew clouds
and sun like a gale of kindness. In the darker woods, a haven
in the Stations of the Cross, my nose tickled. The new life returning from winter death was damp and exciting. I kept wondering which crawling green buds would break through the
wild flowers first. And I was singing a madrigal in Latin.

*"Fiat!"*

Then Jesus walked with me through the woods and out over
the broken road, past the locked shrine of St. Anthony.

"On this earth I am a man. On earth men and women are
separated. In eternity they are one," He said.

I followed Him to an outside altar seldom used.

He leaned His hand on the edge. "You will not be able to really explain it," He said. "But listen, and later write it down.
And if it bothers others, let them worry.

"Part of life is sadness and voidness, the separation of true
sex. I, as Jesus, am a man. I, as God, am Three-in-One. I am
the Son. But I am your child, divine and human. I am Jesus. I

lived and I live, human. I, as Jesus, knew and know, filled with excitement, joy, and sadness. So often, one does not wish to mention sex in spiritual matters. But that is wrong. I, as Man, know. Orgasm is a sign in body, mind, and soul.

"Be simple and listen," He said. His long nose, His piercing yet gentle eyes, dispelled fear. I sat on the stubbled weeds.

"I am in the Trinity, the man-woman. There I am the one Priest. But I came to time, to earth, to be the Servant, to be human, to save all. I could not be everything in that life. Even I, the Suffering Servant, could not be a womb-maker. To be human separates true sex. I had to accept to be a waiting-to-be child, to be a man. Received, nourished, and brought forth by a woman.

"Who is more lonely? The woman, who is filled with know-ingness? Or the man, who can only bring forth and fill the receiver—hoping.

"Mary. My mother. My virgin. My daughter. My bride—the first whom I could save, before she was even born—see, you can understand it all. But, in time, I had to be only a man-to-be, living through the void, conceived through the Spirit, born after nine months. I had to know the suffering of being only a man, separated from the Oneness. Sex is part, on this earth, of the separation of body-love.

"My heart was—is—always lonely on earth. I, the High Priest, knew it at the Last Supper, giving My all. My body. My own blood, to those who did not really understand. What a void, what a cry—the Sender, hoping for a receiver."

The wind blew over the sun and clouds as He stared at my eyes.

"Pray for priests," He said to me. "My priests, with Me in them, are the loneliest of all, if they really understand. Pray for them in their inner souls. Oh, April, pray, for they do not always remember what I am doing. How lonely and hurt some are! See these priests who do not touch eternity and time at the Consecration. It is not their fault for being human, that they are separated at times.

"I am the Man of Sorrows—waiting, hoping for a response."

He smiled. "In the separation of life, women do understand more. They know irrationally the joy of fullness. Men know the strength, and their yearning is of unsureness to know if the seed will come forth in the harvest. Sweet-sadness in body, sweet-sadness in mind, sweet-sadness in the spirit, for orgasm is separated from gestation."

He looked at the unused altar, where outdoor dust and lichens grew.

"Why would a woman want to be a priest in this life? What presumption, dear! I could not be a woman. I could not have a womb. What woman wants more than I could have? Step back and do not let them blaspheme the mystery of sex, the mystery of the separation of male and female. Learn from My mother, understand the wisdom of silence, which is a blessing. On this earth we can only share with those who will share together in prayer."

He beckoned me, for it was time for Mass. I stood up, suddenly aware of not being cold. My clothes were a bit muddy, and stubble was stuck to my coat.

"You wanted to know why," He said. "And you know you cannot really explain it all by yourself. He who has ears to hear will hear. You'll look like a fool. Be proud of it. Now—hurry, it's time."

After Mass, Brother Augustine asked me if I had stumbled and hurt myself on the way over. "Did you fall in the mud? At least you look happy!"

"You could say so! I'm always a mess."

And typically, Brother Augustine conned someone into driving me home. Geisty was yapping frantically. And I was shivering as I opened the door.

With the Easter Seal Center I was in seventh heaven, wonderful people in all walks of life. From each one I had something to learn. Over the coffee machine I met a handicapped woman who drives a contraption in downtown Stamford. She had been mugged several times, and her purse had been stolen from her so many times that she, while smiling, taught me abandonment of money and dignity. From a volunteer, who lived with ESP, I hoped to learn her awareness of knowing the difference between overhelping and just smiling at the right time.

Downstairs the Easter Seal Center had a place to eat, and a large "factory" line, where some of the handicapped could have a decent job, working with dignity. How much I wanted to be part of working life! The whole idea of work is part of humanity. Too often, it is taken from the handicapped, smothered with unreal kindness.

Tom Meath, his book not finished but his work busy and important, occasionally had time to talk with me.

"You need more help, I think," he said.

Soon Margaret Bush said the same thing. "Do you know that your benefits would include talking to a psychologist? To have a divorce is a big deal. Would it bother you?"

"Heck, no! I told you I need all the help I can get."

Dr. Richard Tomanelli appeared more like an actor on the road, nimble on his feet, breaking through wasted time. Typical of me, I wanted to put on the table a conglomeration of pieces of the jigsaw puzzle. I was like a woman offering a buffet with a touch of everything, hoping someone would be interested.

A year later, Dr. Tomanelli could tell me that I was then in need of help, deeply depressed, unable to believe in myself. The more depressed I got, the more I overbalanced myself, a show-off pretending to be fine but falling apart. But in 1976 he simply suggested that, if the group would accept me, I should get into the stroke-therapy group. The only group I knew of was Newhart, on television. I was nervous. "Why a stroke group? I never had a stroke."

"There are others in this group who had aneurysms. I know you've not had a stroke. But we do have the same problems." He caught himself, using the "we" level, much like some nurses who use unreal words: "And how are we today!" Oh, well! I trusted him.

While waiting to be accepted, I saw Dr. Tomanelli another day. Among other things, he asked me about my car accident.

"It's a mess. It's sitting in my garage. But I know I'll never be able to drive again. Someday it might be fixed, but not for me. Even though it's 'totaled,' a very smart son of mine knows it can be fixed. He said it wasn't junk. He's been so busy graduating from college, but he's fixing the motor. He can run it in the driveway. He's working at it."

"April, you go home, call the right place, and get someone immediately to put a new windshield on it. That's an order." He smiled, but he meant it. "I won't let you come here until you do."

On the way out, people at the Easter Seal Center told me the best place to get the glass done, showed me the Yellow Pages, and asked around to see how quickly it could be done. I didn't believe it. But it was done within a day. The psychological lift still to this day shines in my memory.

"I can't believe it!" And it meant: somebody cared.

There are still tears welling in my eyes as I write it now. We can stand some pain. We can stand frustration. But what we need more than anything is a belief in the future. To look at a failure constantly was awful.

"You will drive," said Dr. Tomanelli. "I'll give you a little while to learn how."

When the group agreed to let me in, I sat in the circle and stared. About fifteen people were there with a couple of young therapists. Some in the group seemed unable to talk. Others were chattering about their ceramics and their greenhouses. Physically they used everything from canes to wheelchairs. I wanted to get out!

Silently I wondered: Why am I here?

Dr. Tomanelli had them all give their names and introduced me; then swiftly, thank God, he continued with a question left over from the previous week. I watched.

One woman lived alone. She was angry at neighbors and angry at those she had helped. She was taken for granted and others did not help her at all. She was frustrated. But at the group she insisted that she was not frustrated and not angry. She was trying so hard to be polite, even to the Lord, and her shame and fury were so ingrained in the last ten years that she was stuck in an impasse.

A man with startlingly white hair was kind and helpful to all but hated himself. A salesman, an executive secretary, a terrific cook, a divorcee yearning to see her children who were living with their stepmother, a spinster, a retired builder bored to death, and a woman who had apparently never done anything —so I saw them.

*Oh, God, how lonely the world is! How lonely!* So many of these people smile constantly, and dare not see their loneliness. One woman chuckled all the time. It was false. So false that one saw the fear and the garbage under her sweet smile.

"April, we need to hear something from you."

"There's nothing special for me to say."

Shining-white-hair said, "I'd really like to know about you. What are you worried about?"

In one way I recognized that he had learned some of the ropes, had probably been in the group for a long time, and was partly showing off. But I also recognized that he was really a good man and felt toward me. I knew I was almost ready to cry. I wanted not to. I could see that this was where I belonged. My pride hated it. But my loneliness, so alone with what little strength I had to accept the injury in my brain, tore at me.

"Oh, God, we are so lonely."

"But what is the worst problem right now?" asked White-hair. "With your family?"

Fear ricocheted in my teeth. I mentioned one problem. Before I knew it I was sobbing. I explained the possibilities that had been frightening me, with no one to talk with.

They had told me, and reiterated, that this group was as sacred as a confessor or a perfect lawyer. No gossip could ever pass on to others. In the last five minutes of the hour a couple of people gave me ideas and support. Then it was over. Nobody could talk about it till the next week. I believed it. I felt safe.

I took a cab and went home.

Over the weeks, I learned more about returning to life than I could get in books or lectures. I could not cope or see all my own problems. But I could see the problems like mine. And when we work together and share our love, we are freed. *Love your neighbor as yourself.* The two pieces belong in the jigsaw puzzle.

I remembered reading Dante, seeing a vision of people sitting at a large dining-room table. As I remembered it, their hands were locked. They could not reach their own dinners to their mouths. They were dying of hunger. Then they realized that they could move their hands to feed the person next to them, sharing the beautiful feast.

A few weeks later, one man, whom I call Precise, cried. I had felt so awful several times crying in front of others. I had thought it was not very kosher. I had thought, at times, it was an act, humiliating the patient and putting him in a bad situation. Part of me wondered if the modern craze for psychological games is wrong and sick. Yet now I understood Dante. Later, a new woman in the group asked the same question of me.

"That's all right for some people. But I'm a Catholic. I don't need that. It's not polite. Let God take care of us," she said.

"You're wrong," I said. "One of the problems of the Catholics is the fact that we are told to shut up, pray quietly only between ourselves and Jesus. Do you dislike the so-called modern Mass?"

"Yes. Latin, mystery, and prayer in silence."

"Jesus said when two or three are gathered together—not one. He'll talk to you alone, of course. But He told us the second great commandment: Love your neighbor as yourself. We're all meant to be neighbors: Catholics, Protestants, Jews, agnostics. Wait. You'll see why this group is necessary for God to run us."

Precise-man was crying about his sex problem, mingled with his fear of not being loved at all. To share it with us was difficult. But suddenly I realized that part of his problem with his woman included the dogma of the Catholic Church.

I interrupted. "I could help you a bit. I used to be a theologian. I had a degree."

Dr. Tomanelli changed the verb. "You *are* a theologian."

I smiled sarcastically, but I wanted to help the man. So I explained what the Catholic Church said about sex, and hoped he could relax.

Precise-man said: "No, you're wrong. You don't know."

Oh, God! I wanted to help. I had heard myself using the old terms from a graduate level. I shook my head and remembered a different way of explaining it, in simpler words, making a symbol. I talked. And then suddenly I gave up. I knew I couldn't do it.

Dr. Tomanelli pushed in. "I know what she was saying. Let her try again. She's got a great idea for you. Tell me about it."

Oh, that felt good to me! I tried it again, and though some of my words went wrong, the picture was clear. Precise-man stopped crying and got angry. He didn't want to believe the problem could be solved.

I tried again, and went too far. My mind was very tired. But I felt so elated. I knew that though it would take time and hard work, I would get back to so-called normal life. I felt I was really *myself*.

"Boy, you really do talk," said White-hair. "Man, that's something else!"

It was a pat on the back that I needed.

Precise-man felt better for crying, but he had in no way gotten to the core of himself. For the next few weeks he never mentioned it again. His speech was always slow and distinct, trying to be perfect. Therefore he had little to say.

Then a new woman joined us. She was an unwanted woman. She thought of herself as a discard. The group was telling her she was wrong.

Suddenly Precise-man began to talk in normal speech. For almost seven minutes he worked like a good salesman, giving her a real ego-pusher, filling her with belief in herself. He used every technique of the lover.

His eyes sparkled. Then, as the group moved to another question, I watched Precise-man fall back into his old routine of being nothing. And I burst out laughing.

"Tit for tat. Do you know what we have done to each other? I wanted to help you, so I found inside myself the strength to get back to work. Yet I couldn't. I found myself still not believing in myself. I thought that the one day I could explain theology was a freak of nature. But I saw you today working to help this gal, and you were for a while believing in yourself. Then it stopped."

It's miracles like that that occur, not overnight, but in hard work and time. But the feast is all in front of us.

Small problems arrive along the way, magnified by fear in returning to life. Most women do have to go into the hospital for light surgery. With Alice Carlheim to bolster my confidence, and Dr. John Nolan, my gynecologist, I learned not to be so scared. To have anesthesia shook me with fear. I was afraid the slow mending in my brain would really fall apart. I would never suggest having an operation just to prove yourself. But I was delighted when I made it with flying colors.

"Everything's fine," I would say. "And yet—"

At the stroke group, I talked about wondering whether I'd ever go back to teaching at the university. How does one explain to others the bridge that exists between the rehabilitation and the well? Only by accepting Babel, and learning to translate the language of love.

"Do you really want to go back to teaching? Then, look at the cards you have from your time in the hospital in New York. Reread them, and see what you feel from your time of teaching."

I had the cards in a box. Many of the cards were just the sort of required get-well notes, polite, necessary. Certain ones from the university spelled out real concern. In this book I cannot mention them all. But one I must: Elizabeth Pinder, a secretary, who remembered me with cards often, month after month for years. And before I could write at all I had asked Mary Ball to make a note in the box: Dr. Amos Nannini.

"Were they close friends of yours?"

"No. Dr. Nannini was of the old school, polite, meeting me in the corridor, bowing about the weather. Mrs. Pinder was also just really kind."

"Do you look up to see who didn't send a card?" said the stroke group.

"No. I remember who didn't. But I wouldn't want to count them out. I used to mean to mail cards and forget," I said.

"How many came to see you in four years?"

"Forget it," I said. I felt nervous. "Who cares?"

"Tell us. We want to share it."

"One woman came once. One man came when he left the university and moved elsewhere. Bunny, my godchild convert. Father John came. And, of course, President Kidera and his wife came soon after the operation." I got angry. "Why ask these questions? They were busy. Very busy! What kind of therapy is this?"

Oh, shit! All the first words after my operation came pouring back.

"But you have been back to the university quite a few times. Don't you hate them?"

"People smile at me there." Silence. "I think they're scared. They're like people who don't know what to say. I want to shake them! I want to cry out!" I thought: It's like a disease they don't want to catch. Or else they're afraid to hurt you. It's like knowing someone with real inoperable cancer. They fall back, and smile, and run away.

"So, what do you think you should do?"

"Cry Babel."

"It won't mean anything."

"Forgive them," I said, saccharine sweet. "But, my God, that's not truthful. I'm too scared to say anything, because I hate them. No. I don't hate them. I just hate the fact that they don't know what to say. Babel—help me!"

And then I said: "Who knows? Maybe they never did like me anyway. Maybe that's why."

"Why don't you go up and see?"

When I was ill, Dr. Don Brodeur had sent me a beautiful dried arrangement of a bird's nest. A friend brought me up, and I stopped by to thank him. He is a teacher of psychology, and I talked with him about aphasia.

"My class is just about ready to study it. Would you come and talk?"

"I'd do anything to help others understand. I don't know how well I'd do."

"Will you come?" asked Dr. Brodeur.

Nervous, happy, running a gantlet of emotions, I was thrilled. I wouldn't be a teacher, but from a patient's point of view I could help.

At the same time I began reading books on aphasia. One, by Helen Wulf. I was hooraying—and squashed. It was so good, as an autobiography of aphasia, that at first I could not see why I should ever try to write my book on it. With brilliant images, she was explaining a personal view of rehabilitation. I still praise her and wish everyone would read her book. But after a few weeks, after writing Helen, I began to believe I might have something else to add to the in-depth study of aphasia.

"Will you finish your book? Will you want to be able to teach?" the group asked.

"I will. . . . I think. I don't know. I'm too simple to teach anything but live the truth. And I am so lonely."

And sitting on the front steps at home with the viburnum, I wanted to run away, but the white-pine perfume held me. *Self-*

*abandonment*. The words, and the book by Cassade overwhelmed me.

"Give yourself back to the Lord. Abandon yourself to God. Let Him use you. *Suscipe!* Let go!" I said.

"Will you?" Jesus asked.

"It makes no sense to me. It doesn't! I'm drunk on the perfume of a crazy life You run. I do love You!"

But I am so lonely, I said in silence. And so weak that I cannot even hide it. How much I wish I could be rocked to rest!

I was like an old lady with a large handbag, rummaging through it constantly, dropping tiny papers and secrets on the floor. I could not stick all the pieces of my brain together at the same time. Close the bag and walk, and I felt free and young. But explain why I was doing something, and I'd stumble and rummage around again in that messy purse.

Mrs. Bush, the speech teacher, gently reminded me that I still had problems remembering a few basic concepts. "Nouns, verbs, prepositions, idioms. But you're doing well. You don't have to be perfect."

Jo Moran, my dearest friend, came to New York for a language convention and I stayed with her. "Of course you'll be teaching. But you don't believe in yourself. You're not seeing yourself the way you used to. Giving to others you're great, and you make darn' good sense to help them. But you don't like yourself."

"Oh, shut up," I said as we hustled around Manhattan. "Come and see the museum and the shops before your next seminar."

At breakfast the next day, she got righteously angry at me. "Over the phone last night when I called my Bill, you didn't want to talk with him much. I know he's hurt."

"Jo, I'm getting a divorce. I don't feel right talking to men.

Woman to woman; that's all right. But I'm not a couple any more."

"You're still you. And you're retreating into yourself. You could be very nasty to Bill, and he wouldn't know why."

Jo reminded me of another Bill. Bill O'Malley, a stately, giant saint of the Broadway box-office game. I wonder if there is anyone who doesn't love him. A Knight of Malta, who carries kids high over his shoulders and truly loves everyone from actresses to cleaning women. His wife, Wini Shaw, the movie singer, famous for "The Lady in Red" and "The Lullaby of Broadway," had a stroke with heavy aphasia.

"When I was coming to New York for this convention," Jo said, "you called Bill O'Malley and asked for help in getting tickets."

"Yes," I said. "I was scared to, but I wanted to help you. I wouldn't do it for myself. I'm almost divorced. Bill O'Malley and Martin were friends back in college."

"Do you really think you aren't a friend of his still? My Bill and I and Bill and Wini are friends."

"That's why I called Bill O'Malley for you. That seems safe. But don't you know I'm a nothing all by myself?"

Jo helped me see the psychological hang-ups in the problem of divorce. What would I do without friends! And yet I said the truth too.

"I'm at the mercy of wonderful people. But my pride pricks at me. I'm always at one kind of therapy or another. The old idea of humility, as I pictured it, was sort of choosing ways of being humble. That word I've learned. But *real* hewm— hurts, tearing at the lining of pride. It hits me so hard I can't even remember the whole word! I stumble! Abandonment isn't in the big bag I carry. It's being simple and naïve and scared and reacting to whatever comes into my mind. I don't like that! I don't have a brain any more. I'm just a—"

"A child."

"Who wants to be that? I couldn't ever get back to normal life. Oh, well. . . ."

Jo went off to a seminar. I walked out into Manhattan, and on the way I began to sing in spite of myself: "All that I am," by Sebastian Temple. At least in the metropolis, just as in the lonely woods, one could be crazy enough to be a herald, just for fun.

The light of the day, reflecting in the more modern skyscrapers, makes such magnitude of unnoticed visions. The new material catches not clear glass but shadows we never really see. Radio waves are all around us but we do not hear them until someone turns on the station. At times outside we look at nothing because we are in a hurry. But there are so many things, so many reflections. Do you know what you see? Do you really understand, not in wood or stick, not in words, but in awe?

I used to just look at the streets, the faces, the gum wrappers. But, this day, I ended up on a bench, watching the light clouds of the heavens caught in the colors of dark steam, a black factory, and the West Side river reflecting in a rust-colored skyscraper.

A man was eating sweet onions beside me.

"Look," I said. "Look up. With that reflection I can see what's going on in New Jersey, and the clouds."

He picked his gums. "Ya!" he said. "And you can see clouds here that haven't gotten to us yet. They're from over the ocean coming in. Ya! Ya!"

On a desert island there wouldn't be reflections for us to notice, but they'd be there, too. And where we were, the wind blew the souls, bombarded with silent fullness.

"Sing, God, sing!" I sang, starting off to Mass. A woman

looked at me and shook her head. The tooth-picker was still watching the clouds.

Oh, well. It takes all kinds, thank God.

With Joan Fitzpatrick I talked about my pieces in the jigsaw puzzle.

"My house is too big for me. It was fine for nine people. But the house is running down. To run the garden, to mow, to fix the outside—I can't do it. The same inside. But I've got too much stuff even to move."

With Bill and Joan, I halfway looked at places to move in town. A few ideas turned out to be nothing.

With Helen and Bud Mayglothling, I shared my jigsaw puzzle. We talked about my family and the fact that even the youngest son was ready to find his own life ahead. We talked about my writing and my hope to be able to teach.

"If I cannot drive yet, I must find a place where I can travel by bus. That's one awful problem I have in Stamford. I want, more than anyting, to be independent," I said.

I often went to the prayer group with Joan Gray. A teacher and mother of nine, she often looks so serious, trying to manage things and understand. But she knows God. And when she sees how strange life is, she shakes her head and almost explodes with laughter, quietly. I told her that I thought it might be silly to move but that something was pushing me. I asked for all to pray. And I was talking about Fatima, and mentioned the fact that all those visions occurred on the thirteenth. "It's crazy enough to be true," Joan said.

Chris Golightly and I talked about what our life was for and what we had learned years ago from Father Marius McAuliffe, O.F.M.

"I've got too much stuff," I said again. "Even too many books. What books are necessary? My many kinds of Bibles.

My dictionary. Books on Mary, especially Father John De-Marchi on Fatima. Books on St. Francis, on St. Augustine, on Teresa of Ávila and John of the Cross."

"We're not being realistic. April, books are nice, but if you're even thinking of moving, think of practical things."

"So. I need paper and a table and a typewriter and a stereo and Geisty. I'm handicapped, unable to do anything perfectly. Let God figure it out."

"Interesting. And crazy."

"Yup," I said. "Let's go get some ice cream."

Suddenly the oil burner died. On the Fourth of July weekend it is not possible for burners to be fixed. I had been spending money to get things fixed, trying to keep the house up.

Alice and I were invited to the Fitzpatricks' for a fireworks display.

"I'm going to sell my house," I said. "I'm going to move. I'm letting go all ties."

"Where?"

"I'm looking for a dream. A small place next to a pool with a duck and a lucky thirteen close to Sacred Heart. It's there. All I have to do is find it quickly."

"Are you going to look next week?"

"Yes. But I'm going to a Franciscan commitment conference for a week. There's no hurry."

Not by chance, on September 13 I signed a contract for a condominium. On the fourteenth I finished our divorce. On the fifteenth I moved into a place where I had no close friends at all.

After giving everything else useful to Martin, family, and friends I held tag sales and sent things to consignment places. I got rid of about four thousand books. The house was repaired, repainted, and sold. Without Joan Gray and Chris and Alice I didn't even know how to get to Bridgeport. And I was a lousy mover. I knew how it should be done, but I made tons of mistakes. But I was excited and happy.

"You've abandoned your mind!" said Chris.

"What else is new?" I giggled. "I made sure there was at least an Easter Seal Center in Bridgeport."

The movers, the family, the friends left. Outside my town house, the ducks looked beautiful. The Sacred Heart picture was hung. The insulation was so good that I could put on the records loud and clear.

There was, of course, no place where I belonged at Sacred Heart University, but I gravitated toward the chapel. Two men were standing there, strangers to me. One was the chaplain. The other was John Quinn, a handsome media man in a wheelchair. His face showed intense fingertip knowledge, and he looked like a New York executive who needed three secretaries at once. For some reason, they knew of me and introduced themselves. That surprised me, but I relaxed a little. And after Mass I hoped to learn about a big change in the university.

"You know, we're going to have a new president: Thomas Melady."

Aphasia made a fog in my mind. Peoples' names, always difficult to grasp by hearing, seemed to me almost unreal.

Melady? Couldn't be. I must be crazy. I turned to Father. "Would you write down his name so I could see it?"

Quizzically he wrote it down on a napkin. He really didn't know anything about aphasia, but he was polite.

I read it. "Yes, M'Lady. That's what it sounds like." I chuckled at Father. "It's a strange dream. I wonder what Melady looks like. When will he take over the university?"

"Soon. Very soon."

But some things don't change, thank God. The workers at Sacred Heart—the waitresses, the cleaners, the maintenance men—brought me back to focus. Eleven years of friendship was renewed. They are the backbone of any good university. They know more about us than we do in many ways. They watch us, help us, and hope for us. To really know a place, sit around and chew the fat with the workers. Though proud of their degrees, teachers and administrators have much to learn from them.

In moving, I had, of course, noticed that the parish of St. Andrew's was in walking distance: half a mile. I had partly hoped that I could be a catechist there, but obviously I wasn't needed. I wasn't really ready to work at all. I asked Father Bob Weiss to bless my house, and felt safe. I began setting a pattern for my new life.

Aphasia confused my visual picture of where things were in Bridgeport. To look on a map was one thing; to picture bus routes was quite different. To get from my street to the Easter Seal Center took me about an hour and a quarter. By car it took about twenty-five minutes. Remembering numbers, streets, times, exact change made me very tired by the end of the day, and I slept well.

My doctor at the center was William Baird. I needed to be re-evaluated. Ellen Mack, my speech teacher, would work with me twice a week. Dr. Baird noticed that I needed some help with physical problems. We had talked about that in Stamford, but knowing that I was moving, he agreed to wait.

"I think there's something wrong with my body," I said. "When I look at myself in the mirror, I see that the cross I wear is never straight."

"You stand so rigid," said Dr. Baird. When he was listening

or thinking he kept his head high. But he moved like a good shoe salesman, and he showed real love for patients. "Why are you rigid? Do your feet hurt, or is there something else?"

"I don't know," I said. "My feet hurt. But I guess I'm trying to hold myself together. Yuk."

One of the best things at the Easter Seal is the fact that everyone works together, with hardly any red tape. My doctor explains things, notices things, and badgers me. "I don't know a word called 'yuk!' Use correct words, lady," said Dr. Baird.

"I always act things out, and there are lots of sounds that mean more than words," I said.

"Then, be an actress if you want to. But first think of real words. You're lazy."

To this day he badgers me. Thank God.

Then he told me that what was wrong with my feet had nothing to do with aphasia, just growing old. Menopause changes women's feet. Dr. Baird had a gift of being truthful without crushing one's ego.

Each Easter Seal has its own flavor. There were three things I missed in Bridgeport. The first, of course, was the stroke therapy. Second was decent coffee for sale. The coffee in Bridgeport's Easter Seal is dark in color, which is the best one could say. Transportation was always a problem in both cities. In Stamford I had decided to pay for cabs until the red tape of busing was taken care of. Fairly quickly in Stamford I could go back and forth free. In Bridgeport I never did get transportation. For four months I went by bus or by cab. After that I could drive myself, anyway. There was no psychiatrist in the center there. But there was Marge Scheir, a social worker, and as time passed I gloried in her.

"Are you happy?" a Stamford stroke friend called.

"Great. It's a huge place, but I feel I belong. That's what counts. The charming secretary in front, with the phone ring-ing constantly—another Marge—makes everyone feel wanted."

We're never aloof at a place like that.

But aloof I surely was at Sacred Heart University. I was scared to death, though often I looked as if I was disdaining others. I share my confusion now with others, hoping to build bridges in Babel.

Being made simple, I find it hard to get the right balance of sharing problems. To say, "I need help," confuses people—especially if you don't quite know what you need. Much of modern life is compartmentalizing. Business and work is one slot. Playing is another. But to find the whole person is hard.

I wanted to visit my chairman of Religious Studies. We had studied together at Fordham for several years. He was younger than I, and his discipline was Scripture. He was brilliant.

"I want to get back to work. I wonder how to do this. I know what I used to teach." So far, so good. But I realized I should have started differently. I shouldn't have said I didn't know how. "I'm nervous," I said. "And a lot of things have been happening."

He put his hands up over his head, wondering. It was my impression that my chairman did not want to know about one's private life. A divorce, problems of Disability Social Security, the lists of courses, these do not belong on the agenda. Obviously I wasn't functioning the way I used to. It occurred to me that I needed a course on how to get a job.

I saw his problem. I'd hate to be in his shoes.

I was asked to give my first speech to a parish group in Saugerties, New York. The religious education co-ordinator, Kathy Bunyan, kindly invited me. I was quite good, and it was just what I needed to give me back self-confidence.

"Maybe you'd like to meet Dr. Melady. They're having sherry for the Philosophy and Religious Studies departments, and a few others. Why not come?"

I was grateful.

The president impressed me. He had been ambassador to Uganda and Burundi and was a professor of political science, with a deep interest in Teilhard de Chardin—a three-way vision of life. But at sherry one really does not talk much, chitchat about moving, houses, and so on. It was quickly through.

And as weeks passed, I did not really feel wanted. I had no place to hang up my coat. Nobody knew what to do with me. And I wasn't helping things, either. I didn't know how. I didn't feel comfortable in the faculty lounge. In some ways, I would feel the same for others: "If you're well, come on back in. If you're not, unfortunately, we don't know how to help you. It's your job to stand up and be counted."

But it isn't that easy. The halfway-back patient needs *belonging*. And that doesn't exist at work.

I'd take a bus over to the university. I'd get out some books. I'd look at symposia to come, and lectures, most of which I could not go to because the buses stop at night. I'd stop by and talk with Dot Anger, or Dr. Arliss Denyes, in Biology.

And then I'd end up sitting in the chapel, praying, wondering what I could do. I had just received tenure two months before the aneurysm, and was on sick leave. I had no office, no room. Once, I went out and looked at the catalog. My name was printed under FACULTY. I put it back on the table. I existed. Then I got angry. I got an appointment to talk to the new president-to-be.

"Do you know anything about me?"

"I noticed your name. But in the last two weeks I've been getting acquainted. No one has filled me in," said Dr. Melady.

Quickly and competently, I filled in my role in the past and my illness. Then I said: "I think this university is unchristian. It may be named for the Sacred Heart, but there's no heart here, as far as I can see." I knew I was being terribly angry.

My strategy was wrong, and so was my own unchristian speech. But I was myself, simple, in need of so much help.

"I don't know how to get back into life. I want to. I know I'm not ready to teach. But I could do something. I feel useless and unwanted. The dream of this university was based on love. Love is the energy of God's life, and it should be filled with hope, helping, growing, in wisdom and knowledge. But this place is dead. The institution has taken over. It's so busy that it doesn't have time for helping if one doesn't fit in a pattern. I got this appointment because I know I can get help elsewhere. But I just wanted to tell you that."

Oh, I was mad.

"I've only been here for a couple of weeks. But, as the president, I tell you I agree. We haven't been doing what we ought to do."

That threw me. I shook my head. He went to get some coffee and I told him I was sorry I was so rude.

"I'm interested in the handicapped. There is a White House convention coming in May. Let's see what you can do. I will name you as part of the campus ministry. And I will name you an adviser of the handicapped. In a few weeks we'll get you an office in the library. Let's really see what you can do. Any questions?"

"You gave me what I wanted: a chance to prove myself."

"Are you coming to my inauguration? You do have a cap and gown, don't you?"

And, like it or not, I wept. "In five years I've never had the chance to wear it. Martin bought it for me but there was no place to wear it. And I'm crying like a stupid baby."

And in the middle of joy I felt horror. My dear Helen May-glothling had been having throat problems. After a tonsillectomy, everything seemed well. Then, suddenly, cancer took over.

Oh, God, how strange, zeroing in on what we most prize. For a speech teacher, helping children with their handicaps, to have speech removed? My God, are You sadistic if You love us?

The doctors would just try radiation. Eventually she would have a laryngectomy and then try to learn how to talk again.

When visiting her in the hospital, I recognized her old, beloved statue of St. Francis, and I could not cry or smile. What a mystery! Passing other rooms, I realized something. All people are hit with horror. The only difference is that some already know God. Those who have faith given to them are miserable, with awful pain, confused, and almost punched by His reality. Those who do not have faith have the same problems, but, by God, they don't also have to be truthful in faith. The atheist, the agnostic finds it easier, because he has not seen Him. The paradox of Love in the Three-in-One makes no rational sense. God has such strange ways!

As November came, I had much to learn. I had never known the poverty of coldness. With the handicapped, especially stroke people, using buses presents real problems. At a certain temperature the body reacts with a strange level of pain. At first I thought it was only my anger and frustration that made me cry waiting for a bus. Dr. Baird explained it to me. The stroke side has lost its normal reaction. My left side was fine. My right side, from head to toe, stumbles, and gets frostbitten even in woollies. Even in summer my right side is cooler than my left. I am physically unable to be a stoic. I suggest that friends and family understand and compensate for the problem. Shaking and weeping humiliate us.

I found myself crying, looking like a hunchback, tearing

while waiting outside for the bus at Sacred Heart. Several times, I asked if anyone could drive me home, only five minutes away. But they were really busy. And I had to learn not to let myself be put in a difficult situation. The handicapped has to decide what he or she really wants done and find a way, and not get angry and blame others. I at least began to realize I was a spoiled child. I still haven't learned it all.

What I wanted to do was drive. I had been taking refresher courses. I could brake and park and was gaining confidence. But my insurance premium was terribly high, more than I wanted to pay. Furthermore, psychologically I was still scared. I wanted someone to prove to me that I was in decent health, almost brand-new, and able not to hurt others. Who could help me?

Marge Scheir, of the Easter Seal, explained it to me. In Connecticut there was Officer Harrington, in charge of the handicapped for the Motor Vehicle Department. Usually his job was to find special gadgets to help the really handicapped people drive. There are people with no hands who can drive. Compared to that, I had no problems. Marge got in touch with Harrington, knowing I would have to wait in line. I counted my money, planned for a car, and began looking for other transportation while I waited.

Waiting, I could use cabs. I could wait until the Easter Seal Center had transportation for me. But I wanted my regular speech lessons now, expensive but worthwhile for me. And in Bridgeport, in the suburb part, cabs do not really accept short rides. To go from my house to the university was out. When winter came, I began looking for a way to get to Mass. For thirty years I had normally gone to daily Mass. I called St. Andrew's and asked if there was anyone nearby who might give me a ride to Sunday Mass.

"You're excused. You don't have to go to Mass."

Oh, my God! How can one translate Babel? My reaction was
nasty, railing with pride. It would take me about a year before
I could see the other side. The priests' reaction for themselves
was kindness and concern. I missed the point. I had so much to
learn! But, at that time, I only saw one side of the coin. In my
so-called righteous anger, I hoped that neighbors in a parish
would help. When possible, some nearby did pick me up on
the way home from Mass, and I bless them for it. But often I
was too busy feeling sorry for myself, and I showed it.

With real gentleness, attractive Shirley Meade went out of
her way to get me to the choir group starting. And in late November the parish began special services for the anointing of
the sick. I walked over, and afterward the chaplain went
out of his way to drive me home in the dark after the feast.
Small kindnesses like these bring a brilliant ray in the heart.
Those who live in true love of God, in spite of their faults, get
lonely, with their faith occasionally shattered. I promised myself that if I could drive I would gladly pick up anyone, to pay
back part of the charity given to me.

Through the chaplain and John Quinn I learned that they
were planning at Sacred Heart a regular Mass for the handicapped. It was John who really saw the need. Any member of
the Third Order of St. Francis must see what should be done
and quietly use the instrument of the law of St. Francis. The
university had ramps. They could easily allow wheelchairs.
Melady's inauguration speech had asked for more awareness of
the handicapped. Changes in the bathrooms would be in-
stalled. And letters would be sent to all diocesan parishes in
the new year. The university would provide Mass not only for
those who cannot handle steps, but for the blind, the deaf, and
even the emotionally handicapped.

Meanwhile, I realized I was not lonely, just feeling sorry for
myself, not growing. Franciscans can meet each other. It took

a little time to find a fraternity of the T.O.F.M. nearby. The priest from St. Michael's parish introduced me to Vincent Rollins, who easily agreed to drive me there, monthly, for until I could drive I could not meet our group in Villa Maria.

As usual it was my own misery of feeling sorry for myself. To get help one only needs the simple guts to call. Tony Magyar, who had so often trekked down to Stamford to bring me records from the Weston Priory, lives right near my home. I just hadn't told him that I'd moved. And Tim Sullivan, first my student and then my friend, let me know that he would help me when I needed a ride. I remembered those first months after my aneurysm, when Tim had come to our house to give me hope. Yet I had not remembered him, rereading the cards in my box. Was it pride that made me forget? Tim is handicapped. In the past I used to think of myself as helping him. Reality hit home to me. Tim was much smarter than I, accepting what is true. In many ways, he knows more than I do.

I was not alone. At Thanksgiving with Cathy in Massachusetts, I had been resting. Suddenly I awoke and told Cathy of a dream. I had seen Tom Meath, who died falling off a bridge. It wasn't true. He had died at that time in a freak accident, his wheelchair thrown out through the side seat. Nothing is ever by chance. Tom was on his way back to the Cycons' home. His heart is deeply entwined in ours. What a deep furnace there is in Christ's heart!

As the New Year came, I pondered. What would 1977 be like? What was the parable of the year just past? What did it mean?

Jesus said, "Don't ask for meaning. Just live it and let Me use it. Abandon your mind. My loving Heart is almost strangled with words. I am handicapped by *your* own unawareness. Be a child and stop trying to be grown up."

"I'm sorry," I said. "But I would like to be perfect for You and do things right. Why don't You change me and make me good?"

"I am the Suffering Servant, in the two convenants. Turn yourself, and open yourself, so I may use you. I will hold you and gently I will take from you your sins when you are ready. Pray with Me to the Father and be still."

"Most Sacred Heart of Jesus, show me the way."

"Do you know who I am? Do you really understand? Do not ask. Just let Me love."

I said nothing.

"Will you?"

## CHAPTER NINE

What was my dream in 1977? I wanted to be back riding in my own stirrups. I wanted to be able to drive. I wanted to finish this book. And I wanted to be working at Sacred Heart University. Those were my goals.

Yet I couldn't see how I would make it. I almost gave up. Can you know how scared I was?

The answer was clear, though. "Be simple. Ask for help. Trust in the Lord." Gee, that sounds sweet. It's not. It hurts like hell.

I stopped by to see Marge Scheir. "April, you say you know what you hope for. But get a more concrete picture. Look at each goal and see what broken pieces have to be mended. When you see that, you can ask for help. It's best to make yourself ask questions one at a time." My competent social worker has an unusual dark radiance in her manner. Her quietness drains off my nervousness and gives me the feeling of knowing where the earth is planted.

"I want help from Officer Harrington of the Motor Vehicle Department to test me," I said. "Remember you told me about that? I'm ready."

"Good," said Marge. "I'll work on that. And you might start planning on buying a car. You'll need it."

I stared at her. Why get my hopes up? I thought. But Marge was just watching me. I realized I was wavering, and my response to life would depend on my wish. "O.K.," I said with a grin. "I'll really plan to buy a new car."

"Good! Now, how about your book?"

"Well, for two years I've been trying to write it, and it's been lousy because what I want to say comes out like an eighth grader. But now I think the brain is mended and I can write it—sort of. I want to talk to my editor at Doubleday, Bob Heller."

Sort of? I kept my feet on the ground. Any writer is nervous meeting a new editor. But I had been procrastinating about meeting Bob Heller. Why? Fear had been grumbling in my stomach, fear about what the book should say.

"I'll make an appointment and meet him," I said. "Then at least I'll find out what's ahead." I said it lightly. I felt as if my heart were pushing a whole mountain two feet ahead.

"You're doing well with your speech teacher, Ellen Mack. What do you still have to learn?" asked Marge.

"Problem: abstract words. It's—" Tears welled in my eyes. "It's the last piece I need for writing. And the last piece for teaching. And the same for the university and working on the Symposium on Religion and the Handicapped."

"What's this symposium?" asked Marge.

"President Melady told me about the coming White House Convention on the Handicapped. I studied it and realized nothing had been done about religion. I could see it was important. Dr. Melady gave me fifty dollars to help me pay my cabs, and with luck I will be able to drive before that money is gone. Dr. Melady gave me a desk and a phone in the library. We're just starting. And as always, I'm scared and excited."

"Do you feel you're getting normally back to life?"

"I've got a chance. Dr. Melady has confidence in me. That's a big sign. I want to prove that I'll be ready to go back to teaching next fall." Suddenly I stared at Marge. "I don't think I'll make it. Do you know I don't have enough vocabulary to talk or write a symposium? Do you know that? I'm growing in front of everybody. I'm right on stage, fumbling. Do you know that even in the faculty lounge I turn and ask for help? What a risk! But I'm not hiding anything."

"Are you sure you want to do that?"

"No, I'm not sure. But I have to. My God is a strange God, as you know."

"I'm not sure what you're saying," she laughed. "But you're not discreet, are you?"

At the desk I read everything done in the past year for the White House Convention, questions from transportation to schools, from jobs to therapy and psychological problems. However, people grappling with the handicapped are a bit silent about God. Personally I think it is our own fault for raising those questions. In a convention is it not thought of as polite to tread on deep water.

The millions of Christians and Jews know that the Torah and the Scriptures speak of the glory of God, His kindness, and His mercy. But few of us feel safe sharing with others our deepest questions of God.

*"My God, why? And what do you want us to do?"*

With Jesus we ask: "My God, My God, why have You forsaken Me?"

Too often we pass over the question. But at least occasionally we *have* to ask the question. If not, we're all liars and hypocrites. Do we have the strength to ask God, or are we too scared to say it out loud?

Be simple. St. Teresa of Ávila, a theologian, had the temerity to say to the Lord: "Dear Lord, no wonder You had so few friends!" In our time we would say: "I love You, God, but how come You do me like You do?"

Whether we study the Talmud or the saints, or whether we are simply coping, one day at a time, God gives us a paradox.

The paradox does not give us all His answers. But if we would, at the Convention on the Handicapped, immerse ourselves in truth, we could highlight, for all, the problem of being alive.

We could start with one symposium for the Judaeo-Christian people to look at six questions. Three have to do with the Bible. And three have to do with the clergy, and the churches and synagogues.

One question: How often do we *really* think about ourselves and the Bible?

As an ecumenical group, we believe in God and, in a way, we believe the Bible has all the answers. We believe that suicide is a sin. We believe God runs the world and decides when we are born and when we die. We believe there is no other way out. We also believe that we are free and have a job to do.

That in itself is a lot to think about. Our question is simple. How often do we study and meditate on our Bible?

Second question: Do we believe that sin has something to do with being handicapped?

In our many traditional ways of reading the Bible, perhaps we haven't read it carefully. Can sin be seen as a cause, or can it be seen as a sin of past generations? As the sins of the world? In terms of Adam and Eve? Or in the eyes of a Christian who believes Jesus has taken away the sins of the world?

Those are hard questions. Why ask them? Because in the roots of all of us, those questions are seldom spoken out loud. And this I know. Inside each person there is a hunger to ask God, "Did I at all cause it?"

Look at a baby born crippled. Look at a wife whose husband is suddenly struck down. Look at your friend. Look at yourself. There is in most of us a feeling of guilt, from families, swallowed down and hidden in ourselves—which is wrong!

Question three: Not talking to God is where guilt festers. Basically we need to ask Him, *why?*—or we die with bitterness and fear. I surely cannot tell people what they think by their beliefs. But I do believe we need to ask questions of our own beliefs. Is there any more important question? I do not think so.

That most important question has to help you be aware of what you believe about the idea of good and evil.

Take one day. Look down your street. Go to the hospital and watch. Then come home with a picture in your mind of several people you know. I would use the speech teacher who has had her larynx and a breast removed, the paraplegic, a girl with cerebral palsy, the woman who is senile, the man mentally ill. Now let me list for you some of the traditional answers to God and the problem of good and evil:

Some believe the good will be rewarded and the evil will be punished.

Some believe you are rewarded only after death. But some believe you are rewarded right now.

Some believe the soul is real and the body is only a bad dream. But some believe that only through the body are we able to reach the soul. And some believe the body and the soul are one, and they exist in this life and the next.

Is that too much to think of? Yes, but it is necessary. If you believe in the Bible and your church or synagogue and you still look at yourself and your neighbors, take another deep breath and try again.

Some believe there is no evil. Some believe that evil is just an abstract idea. But some feel it very concrete and real.

Some believe that God can restore the sick, by prayer. But some believe that only by human endeavor can the body be restored.

Of a Christian we ask, what about the Cross? In reading the Gospel we wonder, why did Jesus cure some handicapped and not others?

Of the Torah we ask, why was Jacob handicapped by the man whose name could not be mentioned?

Look in the Holy Book at Tobit, a good man undergoing political problems, helping neighbors. In a time of unrest Tobit went to bury a man, came home to wash himself in the courtyard of his house, and bird dung landed in his eyes. He was blinded. Was evil in this?

The book of Job is even closer still to us all, to Jews and Christians. It would be great and useful to study Job every year and meditate on its questions.

These were the first ideas I had for our symposium. Sitting, thinking, I thought they were fine. But, as usual, I realized I knew very little about anything. And I didn't even know what a *symposium* really meant.

In the dictionary the first definition is "a drinking party, especially after a banquet." The second is "a meeting at which various speakers deliver short addresses on a topic."

I almost laughed out loud in the library. What in the world would a banquet have to do with it?

The pipes in my town house suddenly froze and broke. I had to stay at a motel. And my feet hurt constantly, and though I had bought special shoes, my physical ailments sent me, not by chance, to podiatrists Margaret and Alyce O'Neil, who became my friends, a haven.

"You walk too much," said Margaret.

"I know," I said. "So, too, said Dr. Baird. But very soon, with luck, I can drive. Then I'll rest more."

Enthusiasm and hope can overrule depression. With a goal in mind, psychologically we can always be optimistic. I felt fine. Officer Harrington was coming to the Easter Seal Center to evaluate me. With trepidation and a prayer I met him. Like so many others who help the handicapped, he radiates hope. His whole life was geared to joining us to the dance of life.

He tested my eyes. Although parts of the inner eyes are damaged, they are acceptable, because with glasses I have 20-20 vision. With the doctors, Harrington agreed that I should buy a middle-sized car, heavy enough to not be confused by a shaking feeling. I needed an automatic shift.

"The way you're talking, Officer Harrington, you sound as if you've already seen me drive," I said.

"Why are you worried?" he smiled.

He was there to judge me. And I believed him. With Officer Harrington I was actually filled with fun.

"O.K.," he said. "Downtown Bridgeport in rush hour in the afternoon. Let's go!"

After an hour and a half he beamed. "You're free!"

I kissed him.

Within a week I had my new car and named it Brother Juniper. What other woman would talk to the car? With my feet not so tired, and my right side warmed, I showed Juniper how to get to the university, the doctor, the podiatrists', and the center.

At my appointment with Ellen Mack, my speech teacher, I neatly told her everything about my car. So-called chitchat is necessary for the teacher to see how well the patient is communicating. I did well.

"Good! You've been very well organized."

I grinned. "Now, you've been doing well with concrete ideas. You know opposites: male and female, hot and cold. And today we'll work with abstractions. Ready?"

"Yes."

"The opposite of create is . . . ?"

The opposite? I thought carefully. "The opposite of create is to mush around and re-create."

"Think of another way of saying it. Create—?"

"Chaos! God created out of chaos. So the opposite is chaos."

Ellen said gently, "Would you think of 'destroy'?"

"No! One cannot destroy what is created."

Not by chance, this attractively dark teacher, almost by ESP, grasped my view. Speech teachers of course would never give me an *F* with a different conception of generalization. But Ellen realized I was working with a three-thousand-year-old sense of reality in the Torah.

"I see. O.K.," said Ellen. "But do you want to learn the language skills of the seventies? Can you say the opposite of 'create' is 'destroy'?"

"I don't like that. The opposite of create is remake. In a week I'll learn how to say, quickly: the opposite of create is destroy. But inside myself I will hold on to remembering my vision. One can create a bubble. But the soap maker remembers how it burst, and knows it could be picked up and never really destroyed."

"O.K., April. Back to the game. How about 'far'?"

"How far? It depends," I'd say. "Oh, you mean 'near.'"

"Shallow?"

I pictured a "shallow" place, a resting place. Quiet. Next to the sea. "I don't know."

"Try it in a swimming pool. 'Shallow'—?"

"How deep is it?"

"The opposite of 'shallow' is 'deep,'" said Ellen.

"You mean very 'deep'?"

"Just abstractly, 'deep' and 'shallow' are opposites!"

To memorize that and answer quickly took a week. But it took the same amount of time to write out the meaning of a different reality. Deep and shallow converge. By context, they can be thought of as separated, but they can never be opposites, because of paradox. In a running river the stream is never again the same. And yet past, present, and future are all one.

"Ellen, I'll learn your opposites. By God I will. But by God I'll be sure to remember a child's world and hold on to it!" But to hold on to being a child and also try to write and work on a symposium was difficult. For the first time, I kept hoping the Lord would make a miracle and let me be healed.

"I want you to write, with no pride," He said. "Anything is easy with My yoke if you will not fight with pride. I want you to write."

I was silent for a while. I wondered if He meant writing on the symposium or writing this book. I knew I didn't want to write about Him in this book.

"Do you remember My parable about the wedding feast? I am the Master who invited people to My banquet. Only the good people were invited, R.S.V.P. But they all declined. They were too busy, they had too much to do. But I wanted that banquet filled. So I sent My servants out to the roadways and the fields to bring in the lame, the blind, the deaf, the sick, the ugly, the misfits. I gave you the invitation and you accepted it."

"Oh, yes! I know it was meant for me."

"I alone can clean you and make you presentable for My banquet. Do you know how handicapped you are? Do you know that all people are born handicapped? You're not perfect and you partly know it. I'll take care of you. Just eat and drink at My feast. *But do not decline My wishes.*"

With all the people working with ideas, the symposium was shaping up well. Tom Calabrese, of Sacred Heart, knew Dr. Henry Viscardi. Viscardi, born with no legs, became a special adviser to four Presidents of the United States. He was in charge of the White House Convention on the Handicapped and very busy, but he agreed to come to our symposium, because he realized religion is a major issue.

Not by chance I found it easy to get the best panel for the symposium. The perfect Protestant speaker, Rev. Mark Rohrbaum, happened to have been speaking at Sacred Heart some months before. Rabbi Isaiah Rackovsky had taught me much about Babel. Tim Sullivan, a graduate of Sacred Heart, a working handicapped, would add another dimension. And Margery Scheir, of the Easter Seal Center, could balance the social problems of the families involved. John Quinn would be the moderator.. The whole symposium was dedicated to the late Father James Keller, who had started the Christophers and had been handicapped in the last few years before his death. With the help of the interested agencies of the handicapped, the plan sounded great.

But I was nervous. Writing my speech for the symposium was still difficult, and a bit humiliating. Not being able to type, I went to Dick Matzek and asked for a stenographer to help me. My cochairman of the symposium, Dick Matzek, the librarian, was co-ordinating my work, teaching me, helping me. I had always liked him in the past. But now I could hardly believe how kind he is.

What an unusual man Dick is! I barged into his office the next afternoon and found him typing it for me. I knew why. He did not want to let others know how badly I spell and type. I will remember him forever, locked in my memory.

"Besides," said Dick, "it just takes time. Your writing shows that you're really back in the swing."

"Dick, you're really doing the whole thing for this symposium. I'm just a figurehead. You're great. But I don't feel truthful at all."

I talked again with Marge Scheir. "I'm just showing off," I

said. "Do you know I still can't even spell Isaiah correctly? I get on the phone and I sometimes get so nervous that I can't remember peoples' names?"

"You're still afraid. You're almost unable to see yourself. But you've got a lot of guts."

"A lot of guts with nothing inside it," I said.

"Do you know how angry I sometimes get when you talk like this? Your ideas are good. But maybe it's too scary to get well?" said Marge.

"I'm working on the rest of my talk for the symposium."

"Good. Doing this well you'll prove to your chairman that you're able to teach. How's the handicapped Mass?"

I smiled with real joy. "Last week we were on television! But what's important is that here we all, like me, feel secure, at Sacred Heart."

"What's it like?"

"A community, part of the real Church. We have Mass each week and then we have coffee and talk. As Angie Lazarecki said when she first heard about it, 'It's about time! That's what we have needed!'" I stood up. "See how low I was? But, thinking of that at Sacred Heart, I'm feeling fine!"

In my speech for the symposium I was trying to bridge some of the questions about the handicapped and the clergy, the churches, and the synagogues. Like everyone else in the world, the clergy are wonderful, nervous, and difficult. Some laymen believe the clergy ought to be better than anyone else at religion and then get angry if they're not perfect. We are all in one boat with God.

It is true that clergy do not always know how to communicate with the disabled. The problem may be that they do not think of themselves as being born handicapped. And many also feel unqualified, so they pray and step back. To the clergy I suggest that nobody's really qualified by life. If you don't know what to say, then be with us. Touch us, mourn with us if we mourn, be silent with us if the Lord keeps you silent. Don't feel it necessary always to look at the bright side. Poor Job in the Scriptures! His religious friends kept insisting they knew all about God.

But Job knew that we are all born naked, invisibly marked by God. The physically handicapped are chained, openly. Sadly, other people can pretend that they are in perfect condition, but they're not. And this ignorance of reality forms many barriers.

One such barrier is fear of us, the handicapped, especially if we are not pleasing to look at. There are good people who are so afraid that they forget we are all living temples of the Lord. Another barrier consists of good people who benevolently look down on the known handicapped. They really believe that part of our humanity has been cut. They try to be sweet and kind, but they don't think of us as real people.

Let the clergy teach their flock from childhood the mystery of life. Everybody in life gets sick, and infirmed from a cold, or who knows what will happen tomorrow. To be segregated is horrible. Yet the obviously handicapped are segregated in worship—architecturally, psychologically, socially—as if only the well were human.

At such a symposium, one looks at the moral and ethical problems of getting the handicapped to worship. But worship is not all that is necessary. There should be a feeling of belonging in the world.

There are few lepers in the United States. In his life St. Francis took one look at a leper and was scared. To kiss a leper? Impossible, but Francis was one who walked through the barrier, drank his own fear, and kissed the leper. And he knows the stigmata of all physically handicapped people—the stigmata of being unclean, unwell, infirmed.

Dr. Viscardi, who came to our symposium, was right when

he said each uncommon man is born by God. If you want to be a common man, that's your problem. But God made each of us uncommon, made in His image, free to praise the Lord and work in His vineyard. Take your talents, use them, ask for help and guidance, and move, day by day, to accepting being—each one of us—uncommon.

The symposium was a real success in many ways. From all the speakers, I was learning so much. And for myself, I was so happy, so sure that I was great. Pride was doing a jig on me. I was sure I was going to the White House Convention. Instead I went to Bridgeport Hospital.

I was not feeling well. I started with a D & C with Dr. George Geanuracos, one of the most gentle men around. It turned out that wasn't my major problem, so Dr. Sheldon Weicholz, my intern, began studying the problem. With Dr. James Thurmond, I got rid of my appendix and my gall bladder. Along the way I had a light heart attack and a nasty bout of staph and strep. When I returned home I had to wear a brace on my left leg. Pain was my middle name.

What happened? Physically my left leg was overtired, having taken the brunt, compensating my right side for five years. A bit of old age and arthritis, complicated by the fact that the heart attack made it difficult to exercise.

Happy May! Why did God let this happen to me? The physical problems seemed unnecessary and unkind. But we know it is impossible to separate physical problems from emotional and mental and spiritual problems. Each person is a wholeness.

For me it would take a whole life to understand myself and God. But, along the way, I could slowly learn more of my own core. I had said *Suscipe*. But I had so much more to be pruned. Why did God let this happen to me? Because I had a lot to learn.

"The Lord gives, the Lord takes. Blessed be the Lord," I said, knowing that accepting the blessing can be very difficult. Before the operation this time, I was scared. Pain in general makes me a thin-skinned weakling and miserable.

But, in addition, I was more afraid than ever because I had the idea that an operation with really deep anesthesia might undo my brain again. What a heroic Christian I was, going bananas! Trust? Faith? Hope? I tried. But I obviously am no saint.

"I would love dying, returning to eternity. Of dying I'm not afraid. But the fear of continuing to live with another purgatory of no language skill— O Lord, please: not again!"

"You were right," said Jesus. "You teach others how you are not afraid but joyful of eternity. You often feel wistful for those who die. But you haven't really understood how I felt on earth. You have missed something. You did not see the paradox. Living is energy, as equal as death is."

"I like living," I said.

"Even when everything is failure, with fear and pain gripping on you?"

I shook my head. "But, Lord, You knew dying was the way to finish."

"I wanted to live!" He said.

That shook me to my marrow. I didn't even want to look at His face, but I had to.

"My work was almost done. And I was a failure. But you do not know how deeply I loved life! You've never grasped the mystery of Gethsemane. Why do you think I wanted to die? I knelt to pray and I smelled the evening grass, the stones, the olive trees, even the sandals against my insteps. My body yearned for life. I looked at My own hands and felt them and I smelled My hands over My face. Oh, how majestically earthy is human life! For you it is a temptation to hope to die. For Me, it was a temptation to live!"

I was sitting with Him in the hospital room, a place that seemed almost unalive and unhuman, wrapped in plastic. I did not feel much like life.

"You are God, and even as human You were calm and serene, doing everything right. I don't understand it," I said.

"You are afraid and angry. You're still a spoiled child. You do not love Me enough. So you don't like life."

"Yes I do," I said.

"No. Not as I do!"

I looked at Him. "You said: 'Father, if it be Your will, take this cup from Me. Yet not My will but Yours be done.' But I thought it was just the thought of the cross."

"No," He said. "To be put to the test is to lead us into temptation. Why did I sweat real blood in the garden? Not for fear of pain, not for loneliness or failure. But for being human and wishing to live!"

So in Bridgeport Hospital I learned to love life by listening to His wish.

I am still seldom serene or calm, but I do love life. In the hospital I was, as usual, petulant, scared and confused. My children and friends visited me so gently, comforting me, but in a way wondered why I was such a pain in the behind. I remembered my talk on St. Francis and the lepers—a leper who was often too angry to be loved.

How could I love the Lord, listen to Him, and still be angry and frustrated? I knew why. Jonah knew too. He didn't want to go His way, either. He got stuck in the whale. I had gotten stuck in the hospital. Jonah accepted and was great. But I wasn't. I know the Lord was running my life. He had said, "Don't decline My wishes." By now I understood I needed a spiritual director, and not by chance I was given the right one for me.

Quietly but surely I knew that the first priority was to write this book. To write about aphasia and returning to life didn't seem wrong. But to spread out on paper the mystic level seemed private and unnecessary. I was wrong. I realized that I was only a witness. Obviously, when I write about the Heart of Jesus, that is a bit scary. But I didn't have to explain anything. Some could read the book as a psychological phenomenon, interesting to the non-believers. I had imagined that my family and friends could be a bit upset, but since they love me they could handle it for themselves. I wished I could be beautiful, floating into perfection. But if He wanted a witness and reporter like me, that was His problem.

Yet in the month of June I was wrestling with my own pride. I had wanted to get back to teaching, into my own, normal life. I couldn't. But at that point I wanted to hide, and write quietly. I surely didn't think it proper to also teach in college. I asked my director.

I remember him telling me to go ahead and try; to go ahead and use the talents God gave me and not bury them. Even if I failed, I would know that I tried.

"Oh, come on," I said. "Look at this darn' bright white brace on my leg. Are you sure you're right?"

"You're writing your book. If the doctors think you're getting better, you'd better work on the syllabus for your introduction course." Boy, I wanted to take the easy way out. But I accepted my spiritual director's advice.

What kept me going was the handicapped Mass, the people from that community. I, who had been so darned proud, helping others in the past, knew how totally dependent I was on their prayers, their confidence, and their love. I had thought I loved my neighbors. But they taught me how to love myself more, because they cared. And I needed to be cared for and loved.

Their names read like a litany: Elizabeth, Porter, Angie and Steve, Pauline and Jimmy, Maureen and Ken and Amy, Betty, Claire, Pauline, John, Dolores and John, Virginia, John and Bertha, Fred and Anita and Margot. I've never before been on the receiving end of such a group. And they healed me.

Could I teach? The Easter Seal people agreed I was free at last to work. Abstract words were in fine condition at last.

Dr. Weicholz and Dr. Baird agreed that physically I could return to work, as long as I didn't overdo. Physical gadgets could take care of my handicaps.

"Don't walk too far. Don't go up and down the stairs. An electric stroller would fit the bill," said Dr. Baird. "It's much like a golf stroller—carrying books around the long corridors. It'll take time, but MVD might be able to handle it. At least by next year you can be more mobile. I insist that I'll be the first one to try it out!"

Sacred Heart always finds ways for handicapped students, changing classrooms to permit them to attend. Doug Bohn made changes for me.

And inside myself I was nervous.

"I must be crazy, trying this," I said. "I cannot walk more than twenty yards. Then I have to sit down and rest. I have no office."

Dean Croffy found me an office close to my classes, a fish-tank cubbyhole where everybody could see me up two flights. I hated it.

"Are you sure I ought to try?"

"Yes. You'll make it," said the chaplain.

I looked at the calendar. It was now five years to the day when the aneurysm occurred. Maybe it was a sign that I was really free!

Over the summer, I had finished the first four chapters of this book. But at that rate it would take me forever. To correct my grammar and teach was more than I could do. I needed a teacher to correct my syntax, and I needed a cleaning woman.

"That's impossible!" I said. "Which means it will be done."

At the university I asked Dot Anger, explaining my problems. "Students need money. Any chance?"

"Typing, yes. But while it makes perfect sense to older people, few students want to be a cleaning woman. No prestige. I'll try, though."

"The only thing is, I want someone I can trust as a person. Even typing my chapters."

Not by chance, Dot Anger found the right person, a new graduate of Sacred Heart, a poet who types, a wife looking forward to a master's in religious studies. She moves like an invisible chariot, a deft worker in the bank and in the kitchen. She is also a dreamer. Dot Gulyas is part of my family forever.

For some years at Sacred Heart I had known Ralph Corrigan. As an English teacher he is a craftsman, steering a course to include excitement, depth, and hard work. He was born to nobility, though I have never yet seen Ralph dressed up. Artisans are usually at work in peasants' clothes, too busy to read their own pedigree. Some writers are a bit shy. But, with hope, I asked Ralph if he could correct my English, and he accepted the challenge. Everything was taken care of just as fall opened.

Thirteen years before, as a teacher, I had been a heavy, gawky woman, full of energy, hoping to be good. I was a novice. There were no courses on learning how to teach. It took more than one year to really be effective.

In September 1977 I was again a beginner, and rusty, too. For better or for worse, the first day, I told the students about myself and asked their support. They trusted me and I trusted them, and we began to grow and learn. At the beginning I was afraid that some words would be difficult to pronounce. As usual, it was only simple words that threw me. For example, *One Flew over the Cuckoo's Nest* is a difficult phrase. I'd get up to "Cuck," and sho-sh it. The problem was I never remembered to spend half an hour learning to say it. I'd be sure of "axial," "Tillich," "Schillebeeck," and "Dostoevsky." But God bless the students who helped me learn *Cuckoo's Nest*.

By October I felt more secure. Because I had been ill, someone had decided that if I returned I should be evaluated. My chairman and another teacher would evaluate my teaching, and of course I agreed. For the chairman there was no hurry. But there was for me. I was looking for a stamp of approval. Psychologically I wanted a test, just as I had to prove I could drive well. Every Monday, Wednesday, and Friday I was uptight, assuming the test would come. The noose was tightening inside myself. Finally I asked the chaplain to sit in my classroom to see how it would go.

After class I waited, nervously. Father suggested one idea for using Frankel's book. I burst out in joyful laughter.

"What's so funny?" said Father.

"You're talking to me as one teacher to another. Hurray! Basically my terrible fear was that I might really still be in deep aphasia, thinking I could teach and really being ill. You wouldn't understand," I said. "Only aphasics would know that!" I felt better.

I was happily busy. Following Dr. Baird's plans, I regularly went over to the Easter Seal Satellite for the whirlpools and physical therapy. Soon I did not need braces. I had a snappy cane to lean on. Daily I was practicing my lectures and writing this book. I was also involved in Renew, the diocesan group for divorced and separated Catholics, and the handicapped Mass.

The chaplain asked if I would like to be a special minister to the Eucharist to help him. There are many such special ministers in all parishes. John Quinn was already one. The university needed another one. I felt unworthy, but as a Franciscan I would always be a servant to the Lord. And I was overwhelmed with joy that I would be chosen. What a job that would be!

Yet inside myself I still was full of misgivings and diffidence as a college teacher.

A friend called to chat. "Whatcha doin'?"

"I'm not sure," I said. "Sometimes I feel like a reject. The second string. I wish I was really good at anything. But I'm not. Thank God, I feel wanted and liked as I am with these groups. But—"

"You're crazy. You're great. What's the matter with you? Are you pretending, trying to get too much praise?"

"No. I really don't know if I'm good, bad, or indifferent. I really need to be told, damn it!"

"Did your chairman evaluate you yet?"

"No. He's so busy, I never get to see him. But every Monday, Wednesday, . . ."

That is the horror of halfway back to life: not trusting in yourself.

All people learn to put on a good front, and at the same time watch, hoping to see how other people think of them. Only in the locked bathroom do we take a look at ourselves alone, trying to see ourselves.

But the aphasic and the stroke victim can't really look in the mirror. We have a broken mirror, an empty mirror. We need others to lend their glass and make a frame for us. We can recognize a false frame, a benevolent sham, a fun-house mirror. But, God! how much we need a real picture we can live with, bringing us back to full life. We do not have the strength *yet* to believe in ourselves.

Who did suddenly give me the strength to believe in myself, and brought me into life with a different, new job? The chaplain, who gave to me one of the best teachers of ministering to the Eucharist.

Then my chairman finally came. After the first lecture, he looked perplexed. He said that he'd come back Monday. I had seen his face while I was teaching. So, over the weekend, I worked harder for a better lecture. But Monday, I watched his bent head and wanted to run out. The chairman is a righteous man. Though we had disagreed on many subjects, I knew he was honest, and I felt sorry for him when he said he needed time to cogitate after the second lecture. I was terrified, waiting, for two days.

Then my chairman finally came to my fish-tank office Wednesday afternoon, as people went up and down the stairs outside. He said he wasn't sure whether I was ready to teach, though he was not sure how to pinpoint the problem. He would not let me come back full time. He suggested that in the next semester I do two courses, and have three people evaluate my teaching: the academic dean, Dr. Ford; Jim Wieland; and Dr. Don Brodeur, from psychology, the professor for whom I talked on aphasia in his course the year before.

Students ran up and down the stairs and I watched them. I coolly asked why I hadn't been evaluated two months before. "If I teach so badly, it sure wasn't fair to the students," I said. Then, immediately, I got angry, unable to understand what was wrong with me. "Why? What *is* wrong? Oh, tell me—what is it?"

"It's hard to explain. You use a Socratic way of teaching. But it never quite gets together. You talk almost in a stream of consciousness."

Ralph Corrigan, my creative writing teacher, stopped outside the fish tank, making signs: *Have you finished the seventh chapter in your book?* Using all the muscles in my body so I wouldn't fall apart, I opened the door to my office and explained that I wasn't ready. My body was chilly.

I came back and said to the chairman, "Maybe we just teach differently. I don't understand your lectures. Could it be that the teachers I learned from—Maloney, Cousins, and others—are different from yours? Could it be?" I held on to that idea like a last thread of hope. But, looking at the chairman's face, I knew he was doing the best he could. He surely wasn't being nasty. He was going the extra mile, hoping I could be in the next semester, really able at last to teach well.

"I feel sorry for you," I said, knowing it was a difficult situation.

"Don't be sorry about me."

I thought: Maybe I'm not sure I'm understanding the situation. "You'll write a memorandum to the dean soon, so I can get a copy of it?"

Our conversation ended politely. A student stopped by to talk about an exam. I answered him, turned off the light, locked the door, and held myself together to the chaplain's office. Then I let go and cried as I had never cried in my whole life.

"Oh, my God!" In a spasm, I could hardly talk. Then: "Those poor students. Oh, my brain is still broken! Why would God let this happen! I was a fool, trying to teach. Why did you let me think I was well? That was rotten. A whole semester that was false. Oh, my God. . . ."

I wanted to run away, but I knew there was no place to hide. "For more than five years, I believed I would make it. I thought I was back into life. But it is a horrible lie." Despair, mortal anguish—my guts really felt like vomiting backward into myself with green bile. "It's a nightmare, only it's real. A year ago I wanted so hard to get back into teaching. I got my chance through Melady. And I blew it. I needed to find out what was really true. What's true is that I—"

Slowly, quietly, Father brought me back to my senses. "You have the strength to do that. You are a teacher. You can be a better teacher. And you can prove it."

I blew my nose. "Am I crazy? I'm sure my chairman isn't crazy. How do I know?" In that office there was no mirror.

The next day, I asked the students to evaluate me. They pointed out a few problems in me as a teacher. I wasn't clear in explaining their assignments. In general, they found me stimulating, wise, learning much. Thirty per cent found me a little confusing when I got nervous. Ninety per cent begged me to continue teaching. Jim Wieland looked at my student answers and thought me good. No one else wanted to read them. I wondered why.

Inside myself I was sure my brain was broken beyond repair. Outside, I kept hoping the nightmare would disappear and I kept talking about it to a few other teachers. What could anyone else say? Because, hope against hope, I wanted to find out the truth about myself.

On December 9, the chaplain said, "I've talked with Monsignor Toomey. In this chapel, either Saturday or Sunday, you can be commissioned as a special minister to the Eucharist. There is a special Mass already planned for the university Saturday, and one planned for the handicapped Mass Sunday. You decide what you would prefer."

"To be commissioned in front of the faculty, not being fully sure I belong?" I gulped. "I belong to the handicapped Mass."

"You will be commissioned to the whole university."

I prayed deeply, and conferred with Father Roderick, c.o.f.m., in charge of our Third Order of St. Francis fraternity. I chose the handicapped Mass, where I felt secure. I could hardly believe the honor God was giving me.

The chaplain was angry at me for using the word "honor." Honors are not given like rewards. He felt it was wrong to even mention it to others. But he didn't understand.

The honor God had given me was the greatest of gifts. In *Suscipe*, I had given everything back to Him. Five years ago, I couldn't say my catechism. I couldn't write the Our Father, or walk to Mass. I could not help anyone. Yet now to me it was a miracle. Do you know what He has done for me—Holy is His Name—to use me to help others? Be quiet I could not be. Each day, I cry with joy.

In excitement, I began wrapping tiny presents to thank those who sustained me in our community. I wanted so much to tell my children about it, but I knew they already had many plans set. There were only two days left and I felt it wrong to ask them to make last-minute changes. Almost midnight Saturday, Cathy called, sensing some special excitement within me. She wheedled it out of me.

The community knew nothing about it either. As Mass started, someone touched the back of my neck. I looked and exploded. In eleven hours, Cathy had gathered almost the entire family. For an instant, our friends at Mass were shocked and scared, wondering why I was bawling. But joy reigned. Later, at the Christmas party, to each I gave a special present. I had wrapped a paperback of my favorite book, *Self-Abandonment*, for my teacher of the Eucharist.

I was still waiting to see my chairman's recommendation. A few days before Christmas, I couldn't stand waiting. I asked Dean Ford to get the chairman to talk with the three of us and understand the terms. The chairman explained it again, and said all our future talks would be handled only through the dean.

"I'm awfully confused about DSS and DVR and money and everything," I said. It wasn't that money really touched the issue, but it was easier to talk about that.

"I'll give you full-time employment, even though the chairman feels safer to let you do two courses," said Dean Ford.

"That's wonderful," I said. "I trust in you. But—" I faced the fear in me. To the chairman I said, "You're worried about my brain damage, aren't you? All the tests I've had show that I'm competent. But evaluating me, you don't feel safe. And I don't feel safe with you at all. But you're the chairman. So—the only way to find out, I guess, is to live it through. I think I can prove to you that I'm well."

Poor chairman. I felt safe with the dean, with Brodeur, with Wieland. But I made the chairman the ogre in my mind. I told myself that was silly. I called Brodeur to see if I could start learning some of the techniques of teaching during the semester break. He was interested, but by protocol he hadn't yet been involved, so he had to wait for the chairman to talk to him.

Basically, the question was simple: Did I believe in myself? I certainly wasn't sure. In my own vocabulary, I believed I was going to have four teachers teaching me how to teach and watching me like a hawk. And in the same, inner vocabulary I believed that my ogre did not believe in me and was afraid my brain was broken. True or not, that's how I felt. I sighed and said: "The only way to find out is wait. Maybe when the chairman writes the memo for the files, I'll understand." I looked at life and picked up the work to be done. Seven chapters were off to Heller, my editor at Doubleday. I could not, apparently, write Chapter Eight until I got some feedback. So I worked on the outline of my new course, Religion and the Handicapped: St. Francis to the Holocaust. I was busy. And worried as hell.

"Lord, You have humbled me for five and one-half years. And I thank You. But it is not easy."

He just listened in that quiet chapel.

"My pride wants to run away, Lord. Who wants to be ridiculed? If You want me to teach, let me teach well! Or let me go. My embarrassment makes me cringe. If my brain is broken, set me free! I don't know what is true. I'm doubting everything. The impact is awful!"

"You need to be a translator," said Jesus.

"Oh, Jesus, that's not funny."

"Pray with Me to our Father."

To see Jesus this time on the Cross, asking me to join with Him, asking for forgiveness—to hear Him asking the Father to not lead us into temptation—it was almost more than I could stand.

"For Yours is the kingdom . . . ," He said.

"O, my Lord Jesus, the humility of my Brother dying with us—what does it mean? No wonder the temple was broken apart and opened. The Spirit is moving. You make me scared. You don't look as though You are going right up to heaven. And I don't understand anything."

Advent was almost finished. Meditating, I was still sitting in the chapel. In my hands I was holding the things to be brought to a Mass at the Van Doren Convalescent Home. I was thinking of Mary: *"Fiat!"* Self-abandonment was difficult even for her. For me it was far worse because my own pride is full of pus. I always want things done nicely, neatly, properly, the way *I* think they should be done.

Typically, I began looking at the cloths for the coming Mass. They were washed and ironed, but they looked unclean, darkened by wine that even bleach hadn't completely removed. I tried to fold them differently to make them look perfect. I was ashamed.

Mary said quietly, "The labor pains of my Son, the placenta of my human life, were not unclean. Human life is beautiful. Who should be ashamed? You want everything done well for God your way. But you still don't truthfully understand. Don't ask questions. Follow, and wait till you see a job to be done, and then do it."

I looked at her, and my head hurt. I shook my head, nodding. There was a job to be done? Some of the handicapped-Mass people had brought poinsettias for Christmas, but we needed more. And meanwhile it was time to help over at Van Doren.

On December 23, I awoke and found myself writing. "Let me bend as a reed. Let me be raised or bended. Let me be filled with You, and let You drop away more of the ashes of my own faults. The more You burn me, the more closely the ashes will fall till there is nothing left but You."

I did not know why.

Not by chance, Father Francis Virgulak was coming to teach me about Christology. I, who had once thought I was a theologian, had asked for help. I had so much to learn about. A brilliant young man, with his doctorate from Rome, he was so kind, reopening my memory on some of the dogmas. He was talking about his own thesis, on Pannenberg.

"Oh!" I said. "Aphasia. Babel!"

No one would understand that! Politely, he looked quizzical.

"Father Francis, keep talking. Tell me about . . . time and eternity."

"Ya, sure, if you want."

I was almost shaking with excitement as he kept teaching

me, remembering philosophy and theology, tying time and eternity. And I marveled.

Finally he said, "Does it help you?"

"Jesus had no language when He was born! Oh, my God, I see. He had no language. Yet He knew everything. Cry Babel!"

The words were too great to fit in my mind. All night, I prayed in total silence. As Christmas Eve came, the chapel looked gorgeous: the cross draped with ropes of evergreen and baby's-breath—the breath of the divinely human Baby.

Mary cried to me, "The angels knew the meaning, so they sang, joyful and triumphant. But do not sing that song so lightly. The meaning of Christmas is not adoring just with happiness and light. Anguish and confusion is part of that song. My Child was not who I thought. Sing joy, without knowing why. Accept, without knowing why—in your life, in each one's life."

With others I sang, "Oh, come, let us adore Him, Christ the Lord."

I watched Mary's face and I said, "Mother, you were just a kid yourself. You kept all things in your heart. That sounds so gentle and wise. It wasn't, was it?"

"No. I had much to learn, as all do. Angels, signs, portents, joy, grace—and at the same time doom and destruction and no way of knowing what it all meant. Within a year, dear, I was old in many ways. Just blind faith. That's all."

"I'm not good at that," I said.

"When He was born, I was sure He would tell us what to do, so I could just obey. But He had no language but a cry. I could not obey an Infant. My Baby was the Suffering Servant, helpless. And I and Joseph did not really understand anything. But we could love Him."

I saw Mary, stooped a bit, her fingers rough, her face

marked with deep laughter lines and her eyes opened with wisdom. She was beautiful, but not in the least what most paintings show. I looked at the Newborn, trying to read the message in His eyes. Could it be that aphasia is a sign? Could it be that, at least for me, it is a way of focusing the mystery of the human life of Jesus? To know and not know? To learn in time to fuse eternity?

"It came upon the midnight clear. . . ."

Joy-sadness, the music rang out, electric music that evening by the young, large voices of the middle-aged and the old, and one very new Baby staring wondering.

The same was true that Christmas morning, opposites, contradictions crying Hosannah! In my family we always had a birthday cake for Baby Jesus. I had brought two to the Campus Ministry room. And close to the end of Mass, the chaplain had my five-year-old granddaughter, Ginny, bring the cake before the altar. Baby's-breath and evergreen at the handicapped Mass. Opposites, contradictions cry out Hosannah: the world is new, the world is old, and the only real language is the Word of Love.

During the holiday, I finished marking the final exams and turned them in. I continued on the outline for the new course on religion and the handicapped, grounded on the study of Job. And I continued to work on the next chapter of my book.

On December 28 I woke early in the morning to pray and shook with horror. It was the day of the Holy Innocents, to memorialize the little children killed by Herod, the mothers weeping in Rama.

Babel! The Infant, like all babies, sensed the unlanguaged speech. Mary and Joseph had language, but they could not say *why*. Slaughter, and the Son of God? No word could explain.

Mary said, "I could not let Him cry. We had to rock Him,

soothe Him. We were learning more of the Wholly Other God. I soothed Him, but I saw the horror in His eyes. I believed the Babe was in anguish, ready to wish to die in the place of the little ones. That was His first personal horror of the Cross."

As I knelt I could only say, "Jesus. Son of God, have mercy."

Mary said, "My Baby's face was distorted with the sins of the world. And to be His mother I had to be *strong* and accept His anguish into mine. To let Him sleep."

The Coventry Carol! "O sisters two, how may we do for to preserve this day, this Poor Youngling to whom we sing, Bye bye, Lully, Lullay?" I sang it and wept with mystery.

On New Year's Eve, as usual, I tried to look back at the year nearly done and offer it to the Lord. What did it mean? Unmeaning? Unresolved? No language save Love?

Before 11 P.M., I went to the chapel. There was no one there save the priest, and his mother and father. In vigil before the Mass I let the silent emotion of the year pass through—from start to end. Two wordless questions with no answers. I prayed, offering them to the living Heart.

The priest used "Auld Lang Syne" to sing at the Eucharist. Unusual, it hits the right chord, meeting time and eternity.

"We'll take a cup o' kindness yet. . . ."

Like a mess, I wept. Mary treasured all these things and reflected on them in her heart. But I am not strong, as Mary was. With joy-sadness I cried. What's going on? How can mysticism and common sense go together?

We wished ourselves a new year. The family offered me hot chocolate, but I shook my head and went out in the new year. I can't stand cocoa!

## CHAPTER TEN

In the new year—actually on January 23, 1978—in terror and in faith, against the advice of several, I quit my job. I resigned from Sacred Heart University. At the time, I could not tell you completely why. I was miserable. But I certainly did not want to tell you about it all. And I had no idea what I was supposed to do next.

Two days later, I had my regular appointment with Dr. Baird.

"You look awful. What's the problem?" I thought I was wearing a neat outfit. "It's not your clothes. But I've never seen you so low."

Succinctly I told him the facts. He stared at the ceiling. "How's your book going? You've finished the chapter on '77, haven't you?"

"I guess I have to leave out everything about teaching."

"The hell you do! You've got to write that, lady. You've got the guts to share it with others. Trying to return to normal life isn't something to hide. And with a mess like this, you've got to!"

"Exactly!" said Marge Scheir. "Rehabilitation problems are part of life. And if anyone can share it, you can."

"I don't want to hurt anyone," I said. And quietly I said, "Including me."

"Last year you were the special adviser to the handicapped in the university. But, this past semester, you were alone, without counsel, without strong support. A year ago, you made a big comeback to life. You'd been an inspiration to many people. What horror happened to you when your life fell apart to disaster? What a strange setback! But April, you're not through. Tell it as it is."

"Yup. And you'll know the end when you get to it," said Dr. Baird.

That's true. It is a parable of Babel. In one way it was a classic case of aphasia and its problems. In a larger sense it is a classic case of the human condition in the age of anxiety. But above all it is a classic case of God who writes crooked lines straight and clear for all to see.

Each person involved was good, kind, honest, helpful, and confounded. In a way it is a scene from Job, of God and the devil, human attempts of law and honor and the unhuman wheels of barriers screeching over life. It has a lot to do with prayer.

It has to do with time and eternity, with fear and mysticism, with bishops and God, human and divine. It has to do with loneliness and mistrust, with hope and faith and, above all, love.

The dimension of my returning to normal life was focused in the problems of working in a university. But the same problems occur in banks and bakeries, in parishes and labs, and private homes, in every way of life. Where two or three are gathered together, Babel can take over. I had believed that the problem was mostly of aphasia and the handicapped. But only when I went through that did I delve even more into the mystery of life. I share this with you.

During the January semester break, I was walking on eggs, nervous. Daily I was carefully outlining my new course, Religion and the Handicapped, partly based on Job. I was also writing daily. And, as usual, I was always attuned to evaluate aphasia problems and myself. Two signals caught me by surprise.

My editor, Bob Heller, came up to see me. Like any born reporter, he was interested in Bishop Curtis and Sacred Heart University. At that time, the university chaplain mentioned the 1970–71 synod, in which I had been involved. I had no real memory of that.

"Was I in on it? What did I do?"

A few days later, Father went out of his way and brought me a copy to peruse. I read it, awakening half memories, and I stared at a blurred picture of myself giving a talk.

At about the same time, I had to completely read my own autobiography, *The House with a Hundred Gates.* Friends had read part of it to me a few years ago. But, in January, to answer a few legal questions, I had to read it totally. Again, I felt so strange.

Is that part of aphasia? Yes—and yet I began to realize that the same things happen to other people, not just those with brain damage.

Look in your attic or a forgotten drawer. Look at a picture in your scrapbook, a picture of you in the past. By looking, you are relearning yourself, feeling and seeing new insights of who you are. Your accomplishments and your mistakes tell you a new meaning if you study them truthfully.

Do you remember the story of Peter Pan who lost his shadow? Quite often in aphasia I thought I had no shadow, for it was hidden in the closet. But when I found a new piece of memory, I saw behind my real shadow again, and like Peter Pan, I would test it to see if it fit.

Obviously, deep aphasics are separated from their shadows, totally unsure of who they are. Aphasics are handicapped by real separation of memory. Their minds are inside out, like a starfish, which must push its hungry stomach out through its own mouth, swallow its food, and digest its memory on the way. But aren't we all aphasics, in a way? Some people's memories are inside in, that's all. And it may be harder when your memory is too deeply hidden in the unconscious. But all of us have fear. Maybe some people are really nearly in control. But I doubt it. We're all a bit nervous.

I knew I was nervous, and was constantly testing my memory to see if I was "normal." But I decided memory loss is quite normal, and told myself that several times.

Yet as the days passed I was still worried. I was worried because I was waiting for a written memo from my chairman explaining my problems teaching. Why did I wait for a written memo? Two and a half years previous, my aphasia condition had been re-evaluated as "mild." My auditory modality made it difficult to hear certain sounds. When nervous, I felt more secure with visual cues, as partly deaf persons do. Best of all, I preferred to hear and read at the same time, to be doubly sure. The strain of understanding the chairman's predicament about my teaching made me scared, waiting and waiting for his written memo. Like a kid waiting for his final grade, I was trying to be calm but I wasn't calm.

I had believed I was through with aphasia, but I wasn't feeling sure.

One of the problems in Babel is the need for the disabled to have a complete list of resources. I, thank God, was then able to read. With my monthly check from Disability Social Security that fall, I noticed a bulletin had been included on help for disabled persons from the Division of Vocational Rehabilitation, sponsored by the State Department of Education. I wasn't sure I needed help, but for the heck of it I wrote to the district in Bridgeport. After a bit of red tape, I met Pam Pratt, a tall, refreshing gal with style. She was to be my counselor. I explained proudly that I would soon be free from disability checks, able to be back working full time once again. I was sure I had a job at last. But physically maybe I could get some help, as Dr. Baird suggested.

I was surprised to learn that in 1920 the federal government began subsidizing rehabilitation, a program that has been in effect in Connecticut since 1927. It is so well organized that in five districts anyone can get help within a few miles of one's home. How do people learn about this? Some doctors steer their patients, but frankly few doctors have time to read everything. How, then? By various agencies, by newspapers, bulletins, and word of mouth. Part of it is the fast pace of time.

And part of it is Babel, at least for me, with that damn' pride. In January, I was so afraid, believing my brain broken, I was not thinking of telling Pam Pratt. As nearly as I understood it, DVR was for people who wanted help from the State Department of Education. Education, I didn't need. Either I was a capable Ph.D. or I was crazy, so . . . what could she do?

The one place where I felt completely safe was at the Easter Seal Center. At one satellite of the center I sat in my whirlpool bath, talking with Terri Henderson, my physical therapist. A meek-looking girl, she has the strength of a little lion, and vibrates trust to her patients. I trusted her, knowing that she would not look down on fright, dismay, or tears.

"Halfway back to life is so strange," I said. "What is 'real life' like? Is it only the sick and half well who accept us and fill us with trust? When we graduate, will we no longer feel needed? Do normal people trust themselves? Do they separate their inner selves from their everyday lives?"

"You are quite normal, graduated or not. Everyone is afraid at times," she said. "Every day is new, though. And everyone, everywhere is only halfway back as long as you live."

That made me feel good! But on January 19 I received the

chairman's concise memo. In addition to having the three other teachers evaluate me as a part-time teacher, he thought it would be well to have a clinical psychologist appraise the situation. And for the good of all, he felt it imperative to determine by the end of the spring semester whether I could or should return to the classroom as a full-time university teacher.

I read it out loud. Then I started crumbling.

There were only four days left to the start of the spring semester. Before the dean I had promised to go through that ordeal. To quit now was unkind and nasty. But my brain flashed: Get out of here! And I fled.

To the chaplain I said, "I'm resigning."

"Why are you doing that? You already decided to prove yourself and win."

"I sure wish I could. But I can't! It's not safe for me with this stress. In my emotional state I obviously can't teach! I don't believe in myself! I *think* I'm competent as a writer and as a teacher. But I really don't know."

"We had all this taken care of. Why are you changing your mind? April, come on. This doesn't sound like you."

I saw the terror almost ballooning out of my mouth. I believed that my brain was so damaged that while I thought I was well, I hadn't known the truth. I meant it. And at the same time I wondered why I was saying this. "Oh, God. I need help!"

At home I listed possibilities.

"Who can help me?" I wrote.

"My family? My children are away, save one who is a student in the university." *Cross it off.*

"My brother? Working for more than a year on a book on Lee Harvey Oswald. A managing editor with a tight deadline." *Cross it off.*

"Close friends? Outside the university none would understand. In the university? I have no close friends there.

"Get the AAUP? Get a lawyer? Have a teacher's court? Of
course not! That's not my way."

If I had the strength to believe in myself I could laugh it off,
and not be worried.

"Give it to God, and get going," I said. But, this time, it felt
different.

I tore up the sheet of paper in tiny pieces. Then I prayed. I
meditated. I reached silence, open to the Trinity.

When I returned, however, I was again confused. I believed
I was supposed to resign, and also to look into myself.

I remembered that I had always been unsure of myself, even
before I was sick.

Even in boarding school, in my early teens, I was too scared
to try out for the debating team. I wanted to, and just before
tryouts I'd quit. In college I was the editor of the newspaper,
but I couldn't debate even there. I could rise to a question. But
to fight, to be angry, always closed my mouth with fear. I, who
looked confident, was very damn' timid. Why did I finally become a good speaker, after college? Because I wrote books that
my editors thought were great. With their proof, I believed in
myself. But when, years later, I went to graduate school, I was
afraid again. Writing papers I was safe, because my marks
were good. But each semester a group of profs had to evaluate
the candidates. I would walk into the room and forget everything. God bless Father Berry, a prof who was smart enough to
believe that I couldn't really be stupid. Much like Officer Harrington, Father Berry let me relax, and filled me with optimism
and trust, before asking me questions. Many young children in
school flunk exams. What is the matter with them? They need
love and trust to bloom. And when they don't get basic love,

they are nasty kids, acting like spoiled brats, determined to prove themselves failures.

Was I being a spoiled brat, hoping to be saved with love? At my age?

Without saying it in so many words, I was totally asking for a sign. My life was based on Caussade's *Abandonment to Divine Providence*. And one thing you don't do with that is to ask for a sign. Yet I was doing that. I knelt again. "Where in hell is this terror coming out from me? You ask me to look in myself. I love You and yet I am a skeptic by nature because I do not believe in myself. Don't be angry at me! But tell me. . . ."

But what I was asking through Him was a much deeper answer. Whether you are a practicing Christian or Jew, or whether you use a different phrase for your ultimate concern, at special times you will be open to your core. For those who are returning from rehabilitation, this will be understood the more quickly. A question will trigger a response, for example, about a job. On a deeper level, wordless questions are involved: money, marriage, human love, usefulness. Wordless, but the real riddle stares at you with the question of this age.

"Who am I, and *why*? And am I real?"

Part of my cry was not about teaching or resigning. It had to do with writing this book. For the past year, I had often been filled with terror because I kept having overwhelming awareness of Jesus and His living Heart, and I was afraid I might be making it up. For that, there is no lie detector to answer what is true. Only faith can answer it. To believe in God at a distance is fairly easy. To believe that He loves us so intimately often made me weak, afraid of overstepping the holy. The simplest way, the only way, was to just pass everything on to my director and let it be.

To comfort me, the Lord sent me a real sign in November of 1977, when a bishop, Aldo Mongiano, I.M.C., of Brazil, came to my front door. I had met him in Fatima, Portugal, some twenty years ago, when he was rector in the house of the Consolata Missionary Society. We had not seen each other since then. It is one thing to read about mysticism and the gift of discernment, but quite different to witness it. Bishop Aldo told me what I had seen, what I was writing, and, even more, what I will not write. He insisted that I must finish the book quickly. Then he returned to Brazil, saying he would pray for me.

With the most important people I love, I shared my excitement. A few did believe me totally. Others who love me were quite normally perplexed and a bit worried.

I wanted my spiritual director to talk to Bishop Aldo. But he had the perfect answer for me: "By their fruits they shall be harvested. I do not know. I do not know your Bishop Mongiano, and if I did I still would not know. Doubting Thomas is necessary."

In November I was content. But by December? Maybe you can understand why my chairman's evaluation shook the whole of my being. If, after aphasia, I couldn't teach well, how dare I write about seeing God? Was I capable, or was I a very sick person? Oh, God, I was scared!

Like all Catholics, I believe that the sacraments mean that there is a real supernatural strength of God on this earth, which makes no perfect sense, except in faith to God, the Father. I believe God made every person on earth. I also believe that through baptism and the other sacraments God uses this supernatural strength. I believe God ordains certain men to use this because they were trying to be His servants.

As I see it, every person born is His, like it or not. He uses us, in spite of our own will. We are all messengers, errand runners, at times. "Off call," we are quite human, full of faults, chatting, fighting, playing. But when the Master calls us, knowing it or not, we are "on call." We are living actors in various roles: sometimes the stars, or the butler or maid, or the janitor—or whatever fills the bill. Our own freedom is up to us to accept on faith. But the part in the play He will use us for is predestined, whether we know it or not. At times it seemed to me the Lord was using us, using Father, using me "on call," understanding what was happening. But at times, as if "off call," I was moving in a fog. I hoped Father would guide me, but I often felt we were on two different peaks in a mist.

Early in January, the mystical cloistered nun and her spiritual director asked if my spiritual director and I would come for a meeting. Father kindly agreed. I silently hoped I could get an older, wiser director, which would make it easier for both of us. Friends we were. But the problems of the university and myself seemed too confused.

"You two belong together," the nun said to me later.

"I think He sent you both to prove your fidelity to what each sees and does," said her spiritual director.

Can you imagine how I felt? Confused.


As January went on, I tried to be cool and collected. My director was right. "Accept the challenge, take the advice of your chairman, and quietly grow. If you have faith, you should be joyful and in peace."

And I was joyful when I was in deep prayer.

But when I was coping with moment-to-moment life, though still praying as I usually do while working, talking, or listening, I was often filled with fear. And for that I did not know why. That scared me more. Reading the face of my spiritual director, I saw the same question: "If you believe, why are you so overwrought? That doesn't make sense."

For the first time I really began to understand the command: "Love your enemy." Up to then, I would have sworn that I had no enemy. And, in a way, of course we who believe in God have no enemies because His love overcomes everything. Yet on another level, we do have "enemies," people sent to strike at us so we can see the truth. God bless the "enemy" who clearly pinpoints the problem at hand.

In a way, my chairman of Religious Studies was my good "enemy." He could have just pretended I was competent as a teacher and looked the other way. He didn't, thank God.

One piece was missing in the puzzle, the piece of terror within me. At that time, I could not understand why. All I knew was that I had to live through it and later explain it to others. But, in the meantime, I would look like a fool.

"My Lord, You have said to me that I must resign. Are You sure? I mean, am I making this up? Am I being a spoiled child again? Maybe in Your parable I am the one who is growing thorns!"

"You must resign," He said.

With no proof, no understanding, no sign, and no real reason humanly, I staked myself in total faith. I knew I was surely going to be a failure, and I hated it. I told Father.

Alone I wrote out my resignation. The letter was not tactful, or smart. It wasn't God writing the letter, but I. And I was confused and miserable.

Dear Dr. Melady,

I hereby give you my resignation as a teacher at Sacred Heart University.

Originally, I agreed to go through another semester, as recommended by my chairman. In a way, I wish I could go through this ordeal. But I have to take care of myself, and I do not have the strength or time for this stress. I realize now the scene is unreal.

I'm a good teacher and a good writer. To be observed, to get four teachers to watch over me, to get a clinical psychologist to advise the situation is almost obscene. I do not need to be evaluated and observed at Sacred Heart.

I will always be teaching. I believe in myself. To teach here I would have to be free and clear, with no strings attached.

To resign—to give up tenure—gives the answer.

I thank you for your kindness and insight in the past. A year and a half ago you gave me a way to get back into life and prove myself. You filled me with confidence, and I needed it.

I belong in the handicapped Mass. Mass is part of my life, and I shall worship in the chapel. I honor you for your dream, and pray for you through the living Sacred Heart.

For three days, the near blizzard kept us all at home; I talked by phone to five people involved. On Sunday, after Mass, I did give my letter to Dr. Melady. I was sad, but I believed I had made the right decision. It was, not by chance, the anniversary of my father's birth. I was at peace—for that one day.

But noontime Monday, as usual I was heading for the chapel. There, in the corridor, Dr. Melady stopped me. He asked me to reconsider. He said he would give me a week to think about it.

To stand in the corridor can be a happy time: a "Hi," a nod, a sign of security. But it can also be a time of insecurity, of half-heard words. I was so insecure that my head spun. After Mass I turned to two priests there:

"I thought it was finished. Now what do I do?"

"You were right to resign. I believe in you," said Father Philip O'Shea.

"You were wrong to resign. You should return and prove yourself. I believe in you," said the chaplain.

"I believe in you?" Oh, shit! There was no other language I could use as I stood in a little corridor. I could not even remember how to say "euphemism." If the president wanted me to reconsider, there was point in listening to the same refrain.

For the first time since I moved to Bridgeport, I called my old friend Philip Scharper, editor, writer, and teacher. Because he was also a trustee of the university, I had not felt it proper to talk with him when I was teaching there. But, having resigned, I felt safe to ask for his advice. He suggested that in the Oxford and Cardinal Newman way I should get together all involved in my resignation to pray and ask them to give me guidance.

For some reason, his idea filled me with fear. It sounded so sensible. My life was in jeopardy. I should be able then to ask the wisest people, interested in me, to get together to help me. Apprehensively, I phoned Dean Ford, and explained Scharper's suggestion. Dr. Ford reminded me that instead of resigning I should have taken a leave of absence. I reminded him that I believed I would have to come back to the same problem. Ford said he would indeed try to get everyone together.

One man decided the meeting could not be held.

And Babel took over.

I learned one thing. Like Christopher Robin on the stairs, halfway up and halfway down is no place to make decisions. To me, the first three days were a nightmare, hearing so many different reactions.

"*I think you're fine.*" . . . "*I think it's the system.*" . . . "*I love you but I'm not sure if you're capable of teaching." . . . "I know you can but laugh at them all. You're too good for this place." . . . "No, you're trying to be a prima donna. Maybe you should discipline yourself and say you're sorry." . . . "The chairman's no good."*

Trust? I couldn't trust any of them, because they could not trust themselves. I wanted to disappear.

Then I was told that I was causing problems for others, that I was hurting the good name of my chairman by talking too much.

At the moment I hated hearing those words. I wasn't being fair to the chairman. I called him. I tried to assure him that I believed he was in a bad situation and I said I was sorry for whatever I did that was wrong. But I began crying. In kindness, he said he would ask Dr. Melady not to ask me to reconsider any more, but close it, and accept my resignation. "Don't make any more phone calls," he said. "Rest."

I hung up the phone. The silence was deafening. I saw no mirror. I prayed.

"What is true? What is not? Am I crazy? Hide me or heal me, but do not leave me in limbo. Fix my brain or take it all away."

Again silence.

I got some coffee and sat in the dining room. And for the first time in my life, I was tempted to suicide.

"Except . . . I believe in You and Your Name."

I went upstairs and prayed again: *Jesus, Son of God, have mercy on me!* Up and down the stairs I went.

Terror filled the house.

"I want to kill myself, and I will . . . *not!* O God, my God, why not tell me who I am? Why do I say this? Why do I want to disappear?"

At midnight, I knew I needed help. My confessor was out. The only one I could reach was Father Philip.

"I've never felt like this in my whole life. Help me. Oh, God, help me!"

"You're going through hell, like everyone else does. You're not alone. Everybody gets that feeling." Slowly he calmed me by phone, and I could sleep.

But I woke in the dawn again in Babel. *Jesus, Son of God, have mercy on me*, not just said by rote but an inner breathing of love. This time I said it with very quiet yearning and desolation.

"Forgive me. What have I done? Help me to know."

"Yours is not to know—but to be," He said. He said it over and over, three times, and I became more and more terrified. All I could do was repeat my prayers, have breakfast, answer the phone, repeat my prayers, watch the windows, say a rosary, and take the dog for a walk.

Throughout the day, terror overwhelmed me. Fear made me feverish. Everyone has his own silent anxieties, but when fever comes, the anxieties melt into one, spitting out strange pieces with loneliness, and human love screaming, catching even "ersatz" love. Ah, Babel, I was hiding my anger.

I went to Mass, wondering if I was sane.

For just a moment I saw Jesus and heard Him say: "Get behind Me, Satan!"

Would you believe that? I would have sworn He was angry. Sweet Jesus wouldn't get angry, would He?

He said it again. In frustration and loneliness He said loudly to Peter: "Get behind Me, Satan!"

And in that moment I felt secure enough in my old way of just talking to Him, friend to friend. And I said: "My Lord, that must have hurt Peter! Why did You not gently explain it to him? You, of all people, shouldn't get angry with good people."

"On earth, I dared not trust Peter, at that time," He said. "I dared not listen to him, because My obedience to the Father was obvious, but it was hard for Me. Each man has his freedom. Even I could not take away Peter's freedom. But of course I was angry. Emotions encounter so many different nuances of fear, sadness, contradictions, and warmth, desolation. To will, to act, truthfully may be hard, but it is sometimes necessary to be angry. Don't you *understand?*"

No!

I should have been angry at God. But I wasn't. Just confused to hell. How strange! As Father consecrated the Eucharist, I ate and drank, so hungry, so thirsty, so tired.

Later, I spoke with Father. "*My God*, what's going on? Do you know how close I got to thinking of suicide? Why?"

We talked together till, at last, I felt safe. But as I got into my car to go home, terror took over again. Inside myself, I knew I could not trust him. And I surely could not trust myself.

I went home, and in emergency I called Marge Scheir for the name of a good psychiatrist.

"I need to be put in."

I took a cab, much too confused to drive. Not by chance, the right one was Dr. William Sires.

Lamenting, wailing, weeping, but fairly competently and concisely, I listed my problems. I showed him the memo and my resignation letter. I said I had also been under strain because of my divorce and Martin's new marriage. I told him about my book, and about aphasia. I said my mind was broken.

"You're very sane," said Dr. Sires after an hour. "You have been going through a terrible trauma. But you're all right."

I trusted him. Why? Because he would not give me a tranquilizer, let alone put me in the hospital. I decided he must think I'm sane because he agreed what I'd been going through was horrible.

"Will you come back to see me tomorrow, to make yourself feel sure?"

I agreed. "I guess I'll call my daughter to pick me up. You know, I expected I'd be sent to the hospital, or the mental home. Sounds silly, but I hadn't made any other plans."

I called Cathy. I hadn't shared any of my mental anguish with her. I suppose it wasn't fair, but at the time I could not even understand myself. I wasn't thinking, just being. "Forgive me," I said to Cathy when, for the first time in weeks, I could smile with her and little Ginny. "The whole time has been unreal. I went to see this doctor. For somebody like me, to even think about suicide? Or thinking I was mentally unbalanced? That's awful. Honey, I don't know what it means. All I do know is that I feel secure with the doctor, and with you. Don't leave me alone. I feel the way it used to be in the first months of aphasia."

April Marie Ginny Sue gave me a big hug. "I like you, Gramma."

As a crisis passes, real talking isn't the first answer. I was numb, occasionally touching the cringed memory, touching it to feel it again and make sure it was real. For a few moments I went to change into comfortable clothes, and knelt to pray.

"I do not know what's going on. I'm sorry for anything I've done wrong." But I wasn't afraid. I felt very safe, though why I could not then tell you. I didn't know.

As the evening passed, another kind friend joined me, talking and playing my favorite game, Parchesi. With Cathy I felt loved, safe as I had not felt for weeks. Our friend even went the extra mile and slept in my living room, in case I might want to play some more Parchesi in the middle of the night.

When I finally went to sleep, right after my prayers, I knew I was sane—sane but apparently useless.

In the morning, talking with Dr. Sires, I again felt better.

"All you need is to rest and build yourself back to life. You don't need therapy. Is there any way I can help you?"

"I want to know all about myself. I think my spiritual director thinks I'm sick. I wish he'd come and talk with you and me together, now or later after you look at my tests. I want to get every file and test on me, physically, mentally, and spiritually, into one place. Funny, the straw that broke the camel's back was my chairman's recommendation that we have a clinical psychologist looking in on me. I felt so insecure at the university. But now I'm asking you to help me to get those tests done again. I've had them done so many times since my illness, and I was angry and scared to have them done again. But I guess I should have."

"I'll be glad to get all your data together for you." He smiled. "I have to tell you something."

I straightened in my chair.

"I have to tell you that in sending in your resignation you were incompetent," said Dr. Sires.

What was he saying now, as I felt fear raising embers?

"You were in trouble and you needed someone to help you. If you were driving a car and got into trouble with the police, you would go to a lawyer. You would know you were incompetent to handle the matter, but the lawyer would be competent. If you had a pain in your behind, you would go to a medical doctor. You would know you were incompetent, but the doctor would be competent. I am a psychiatrist. I am competent. You were incompetent in judging yourself. With your permission, I want to call the president and the chairman and ask that since you were, at the moment, incompetent to resign and had no competent counsel, that you had not made the right decision. When all the tests are completed I, who am competent, hope to straighten the matter."

How simple that was.

"Now," said Sires. "Go home. You don't need treatment at all."

"I believe you won't hide anything from me. You said you'd read the chapters of this manuscript. If I am crazy, hysterical, or neurotic, let me know. I will accept any help so that I can be straightened. Total honesty and integrity is necessary."

"It'll take time to get the tests."

"I'm not in a hurry. I've got to write this chapter to end the book. And I don't know all the pieces of the puzzle of my life. But I do believe that the devil himself has been at work. That's not nice to say in this modern life. Maybe it has something to do with aphasia, too. I don't know yet. But my presence in the university confounded and confused me and all the other good, kind people there. God, the devil, and Job? Anyway, with your help, although I still feel a little shaky, I believe in me. Oh, God, that feels good! For so long I have believed in Him, and in my neighbors, but not in me."

Before getting back to writing, I made myself a large sign:

## "DISCRETION. DISCIPLINE."

To me that looked good. My director had said that to me more than once, politely. What it really meant: "Shut up and grow up. You have a lot to learn."

I hung up the sign.

"For you, *no*," said the Lord. "To be a child is to be as wise as a serpent and gentle as a dove."

"But I am neither," I said.

"True! You are neither wise nor gentle by yourself. But you

are Mine, and I use you. The cloud of unknowing is over you."

"That's frightening. I don't even *feel* like trusting You."

"But you do. Those of this world are trying to be wise to help you and save you, making you grow up. You did that once."

"Oh, Jesus, just like St. Teresa: 'No wonder You have so few friends.'"

"Yes. To follow Me is too simple for you."

"You made me a total fool," I said.

"You are a parable that isn't finished," He said.

I threw away the sign.

"You know a bit about discipline," He said. "Finish the book. The only way you learn is to write: Because you have integrity, you can slowly learn from your own mistakes. And slowly, you will learn how to know anger."

Anger? I still didn't understand that. But, then, quite often I didn't understand what He was saying.

I started writing ten to fourteen hours a day.

Within the week, Father, still my confessor, tried to help me. "I'm worried about you. You're sick and you can't become a recluse. I know you well. You should go out and do things."

A bit nervously I said: "You really don't know me at all." I began to be a little irritated, but I was afraid that I might not have the friend any more. "Yes. I've been working damn' hard. But I'm not mentally sick. Yes, I go out to Mass at Sacred Heart and elsewhere. I also in the last week drove my car over a hundred miles, visiting lonely and confused people, taking them out to lunch, listening and sometimes really helping. When people call, I listen and help. Why don't you find out what I'm like someday? You've got a distorted picture of me. I'm lonely, yes. Terribly lonely. But—"

"Good, then," he said. "Glad you're not sick. But I think you need to pray a bit. No matter how busy you are, you should, each hour, make a quick prayer to the Lord. Just a 'Hail Mary' would do it. Discipline would be helpful."

"Oh, my God!" I said. "You're kidding! You call me a *friend?* Your name is Eliphaz." I bit my tongue. Read the Book of Job and you will know what I was saying. Eliphaz was a good man, deeply religious, a friend of Job. Eliphaz came to help poor, sick Job, and he was teaching Job how to pray. He was saying all the right words, much as a catechist would do. But he really didn't see God. And Job did. God was angry at Eliphaz. And so was Job.

I couldn't figure out why God let us get into such a situation. *Say a Hail Mary?* In thirty years, I rarely missed daily Mass, and usually through illness. For twenty years as a Franciscan Tertiary, I daily use my breviary, and Mary is part of my life. I pray, meditate, and contemplate hours at a time. *God, who's nuts?*

I stared at Father. Then I said, "It isn't your fault." I called him Eliphaz because maybe he wouldn't know how angry I was at him. "I cannot trust you—yet. I love you, but I dare not trust you. Why? I don't know yet."

In between writing, I often visited other aphasic friends, especially those halfway through rehabilitation. Mr. Z. was having problems with his job. I love him, and he really trusts me. He is a godly man, who would give his best shirt to a stranger, the one who tells jokes, caresses a rose, visits the lonely, and *listens.* He is also an ornery man, often smiling because he is scared, saying little when he is nervous. Just a normal aphasic!

But, that day at lunch, I suddenly saw how angry he was—anger almost like green pus lying inside himself. Smiling, he was angry not only at the world and at his boss but also at God!

How delightful when we learn our mistakes by helping our friends! I tried to explain it to Mr. Z.

"Oh, no," he said. "I'm not angry at God. I couldn't be. He had a reason for my problem, and all I have to do is accept it. He is kind, and I love Him."

"Do you *ever* get angry at Him?"

"No."

"In writing my book, I learned how to be angry at Him. My problem is a bit different. I am afraid to get angry at my neighbors and my friends. The more I love them, the more I'm afraid to be angry. It's the same problem, though. You get very angry at some people and show it."

We made an appointment with Z.'s boss. And I drove home, praying for guidance.

I felt sort of safe getting angry at God, though truthfully I hadn't been quite happy for the past few weeks. But He had been saying that I should get angry.

"O.K., Lord. Teach me how. Should I take lessons, take a course on hating people? Come on! That's unreal."

"Yes," He said. "Get angry."

And suddenly I drove off the road and into an icy ditch. I, who thought I was a Christian, was—damn it—angry at lots of people. I hadn't really been truthful at all. I had been a fraud.

"No," He said. "Not a fraud. Just afraid."

A truck stopped to see if I needed help. I waved, and drove home. Inside, I took the phone off the hook and started talking to myself out loud. Could it be that I was buying human love, not being truthful at all? To people with whom I am not emotionally or personally involved, I was very good as a mediator, an instrument of peace, letting God work through me. But what about people I really cared for? Was I afraid to lose them? I wondered.

"Pick one person and get angry."

It took me about half an hour just to choose which one to pick—half an hour because I would start to grab one and discipline myself into pretending I wasn't really angry at him. In the end I chose the man who had been my spiritual director. I tried to list all the things that annoyed me. That was hard, because, typically, I mentally made excuses for him. But I stuck to it. Instead of praying for him, I tried to dissect him.

When I heard the noise of the phone, I thumbed my nose and went into another room. I tried to act out my fury not with words but by sounds. I wasn't good at that. I tried harder. I mimicked my anger at his unawareness of my need. I almost quit, but then I noticed Roget's Thesaurus in the bookcase. I looked him up under "imbecility" and wrote down every word that described him. "Incompetent, half-baked, muddleheaded, obtuse; idiot, oaf, weakling; swayed, unreliable; ignoramus." I was having fun using these incongruous words.

I stood up and tried harder, pretending that I meant it. And finally, at last, true emotion came pouring out of me. Noisily, shaking in my abdomen, I vented my frustration. Wow! I hated what he had done to me, and it felt good. There was real joy in me. I really loved him. What I hated was my own inability to react in human anger at a situation. When I awoke I hung up the phone in the kitchen, drank some coffee, and realized two things: it would be hard work to look in on myself, flushing out my hidden anger, and yet truthfully I could see what a pain I had been to him, too.

For the next two days I was on retreat, praying and meditating on "A. H.!": Anger and Hate. As an exercise, on one page I listed people, not only people I know but also ones like the kids that throw rocks at the ducks in the pond and the neighbor who calls by phone and complains about the dog and never gives his name. On another page, I wrote words that I found to be the best descriptive words in the Bible.

"Hypocrites. Vipers. Gnashing of teeth." Jesus, who loved everyone, knew how to use anger. Sarcastic? He was almost sarcastic at the garden when He found his friends asleep. "Rest, sleep well!" He, Who is Truth and Love, knows what life is like. Like St. Peter, I have a lot to learn. Like Eliphaz, I hadn't seen the whole truth. But I was on my way.

Since then I've asked psychologists and social workers about this technique. It certainly isn't a new idea. I guess I was the last to learn it. It was a useful and obvious way of opening up anger. There have been tons of books on that. Perhaps my problem was that I didn't dare be "unchristian." What a laugh! I was a fool, as usual, but the breakthrough was good for me at the right time.

Personally, the trauma of my resignation from the university made sense. While I did not understand the whole picture, I knew that I had been miserable without knowing how to be angry. I wondered if that anger had something to do with aphasia.

And, as usual, I was drawn to the chapel for daily Mass and Sunday Mass.

Two days later, driving up for an appointment with Mr. Z. and his boss, I was outlining our problems, the blind helping the blind. With prayer I hoped I could help this great aphasic keep his job.

I had had a chance to observe Mr. Z. at work. When relaxed, he worked well. But when he got nervous, especially when the vice-president stood listening to him, Mr. Z.'s words were strange. By then I had learned the lingo of speech pathologists. "Perseveration" was a sign of problems in aphasics, repeating phrases or sentences when the brain was uptight. "Digression" was a sign, when the aphasic got off the topic. Like me, Mr. Z. was often scared in a hostile environment.

The boss proved charming, and though he knew nothing about aphasics, he was interested in grasping the problem. The boss really wanted to help Mr. Z. But there were many unasked questions. Then we got to the immediate case, the question of whether Mr. Z. should or could continue working at this company.

Listening to the boss, I was suddenly amazed. He was digressing from the subject! Under strain, the boss was repeating phrases, and even whole sentences! Babel? By God, I got the idea of translating his worries. I listened to his clues, and I realized the issue was not how to help Mr. Z. be rehabilitated. It was just a problem of human beings who were caught in a bind.

Picking at the clues, I saw it clearly: the vice-president was a fine and important genius who had not been feeling well and who hadn't enjoyed Mr. Z. before his stroke. Mr. Z. also hadn't liked the vice-president. Mr. Z. was afraid he would fail returning to life. And the vice-president was also afraid about his failing. And the boss was also scared. If he had to choose, he would definitely fire Mr. Z., rather than lose the vice-president, whom he needed. Was there room for compromise?

This boss had plenty of time to talk with us together, because he wanted to do what was best for all. With them, I used the trauma of my resignation to translate human life. Did a miracle occur? No. But there was a real beginning. Maybe in the end Mr. Z. might prefer working elsewhere for the good of all concerned. The boss would also help him find a new job. In time my friend Z. might be able to release his own personal anger at life, and also be free of some of the anger at the vice-president. But, either way, there were in that room hope and peace that flattens mountains.

Driving home, I marveled that their problem was, for the moment, resolved. Mine, however, was not.

In resigning, I was only interested in knowing whether I was crazy or not. But when I finally agreed with Dr. Sires to get a psychologist to test me, I was furious! Why didn't anyone explain what I would lose from the university? Pam Pratt came to my rescue.

"You needed an agent!" she said. If I had asked her what to do with the chairman's memo, she could have helped me and probably none of this would have happened. Now, to pay for my testing, DVR would pay for any help necessary.

When the tests were done, the results showed me still lacking "social judgment" in handling business problems. But that wasn't very high on my list of priorities right then. My standing before God was. And, of course, if one believes in self-abandonment, one does not need any agent except God.

Was there any marked change in my completed tests? No. If anything, my intelligence level tested even higher than last time, getting more "intellectual" all the time. Still mending.

But there was one large factor I had never understood.

After listening to the psychologist, I asked the one question that had bothered me for those past months. "Why was I so scared?"

"Your fear is physical—physical with the brain. Didn't you know that?"

"No!"

"Understand it carefully. Just as you need three pills of Dilantin a day, your brain needs support in a stress situation. You are handicapped by a physical mechanism. The wires and electrons in your brain have been damaged. No wonder you keep using the word 'safe.' Your brain was telling you the truth when you ran away from the situation. It was not a psychiatric problem. It was a lack of growing up and facing reality. It was physical fear because, having once been incompetent, unable to talk or read or teach, you needed deep security."

"Must I always need security? I don't like that."

"As each part of the brain is mended, you will get stronger. You have proved to yourself now that you can teach in a classroom, and you won't worry on that again. The stress you've been under is fantastic. For in addition to emotional strain, that physical fear was shaking you constantly."

"Does that mean I have to be babied or coddled? That would be a lousy way of working in a job."

"No. Just like the physical problem of diabetes, so the physical problem of aphasia can be controlled in a good environment. All you needed was a person who believed in you and you could call on for help. Even normal teachers are awfully tense by being evaluated. What you needed was strong support, someone believing in you. But now that you are more sure of yourself, knowing your intellectual level is not seriously impaired, you will never have to worry about that again."

Tests showed that my brain may still grow better and better. Damages showed that math and motor skills are not high areas. Physically, I was using too much stamina in moving down long corridors, and, like any teacher, I was very handicapped by not having learned to type. To teach at a college level in my own discipline could be easily handled. I could not teach at a graduate level, because I was still too slow expressing brand-new ideas. I would grasp a brilliant new idea, but to express it would take maybe three days.

But should I be a college professor? That's a very different question. The second time around, I was full of physical fear, with no strong person backing me. I was so hungry for human compassion, so frightened that I could not believe in myself. My idea of a Judaeo-Christian religious discipline was quite different from Religious Studies. Both can have exacting standards, but love and faith do not yet belong in the classroom. But I had forgotten that.

Could something have been done to save me? Yes, in a good environment. In every company or group, I believe, one needs a good ombudsman, one who has awareness and *time* to sense a problem before it is too late. What I needed was not only an adviser for the physically handicapped but also a person who *cared* and could do something to rescue me. To hire a person is to make oneself indebted to the worker, continuing to help him grow. I had been a member of the faculty for twelve years, seven years teaching, five years on sick leave. In a community with religious beliefs, it may be necessary to have an ombudsman whose only job is to both pray and work, looking for the needs of others, to fill them with trust, and mediate. To mediate is to bring together the people involved. No one did that.

As it so often happens, good people want to help others and are handicapped by time. The problem is everywhere, a disease sent by the Devil. The helpers, the dreamers, the savers, are frustrated in the traffic of life. Time moves too fast.

Was I angry? Yes!

Now that I knew I was well, I wanted so much to get myself reinstated. Oh, God, how much I wanted it! I was waiting, as quietly as I could, learning discipline. The social workers, counselors, and doctors made me feel sure that the mistake would be cleared, and the horror would be forgotten like a bad dream.

As I waited, quite often when I went to the chapel, I got very teary when people I did not even know knew I had resigned would ask me why my courses were canceled, or asked what I was planning.

Why in the world was I always over there anyway? God knows why, but I didn't know why.

To the psychiatrist, the psychologist, the social workers, and friends, I answered: I have an obsession—an obsession with the Heart of Jesus and Mary, especially in that particular chapel. I mentioned it to all of them, with no bones about it. Common sense would dictate that I stay away from the chapel, cross, and tabernacle, and not mention it to others. But I had to go.

"I have tried to stay away. I thought it might be an infatuation. I thought it might be a hang-up on my wanting my job back. I go to St. Andrew's. I go to the hospital chapel. I know God is everywhere. But, to me, this chapel at Sacred Heart is a very holy place. I come here because He calls me. And because, quite apart from everything else, I have been called, as a Franciscan, to rebuild and refurnish this chapel. With what little tithing I had to offer in trying to get it painted or refixed, whatever washing or cleaning I could do, drew me daily."

I swallowed. People could read my confession quite differently. They could say I was playing a sick game. Some people could think I was trying to manipulate my unreal dreams, to pretend to see the Lord. It had, indeed, occurred to one that I was infatuated with a priest. Considering the situation, it was not likely. Infatuation was not the right word.

"Do I need therapy, Dr. Sires?"

"No."

Was I still angry? Yes, but not just at people. I was angry at the Lord.

Chapter Nine was finished. And Chapter Ten?

"Whoever wrote a book without having any ending? What do I do now?" I asked Him.

"You're a failure, aren't you?" I didn't like that. "Can you find the balance yet? You were angry and sarcastic. You were angry in despair. Are you yet able to just *be?*" He asked.

"Jesus, tell me who I am and what for."

"I tell you again, child: what I want you to be."

"But You do not tell me," I said.

"When I wish to, I will. Freedom is to abandon knowledge and just be. To act and react, just loving Me. Your friend St. Augustine said it right: 'Love God and do what you will.'"

I guess one of my worst problems is trying to understand. It sounded strange, though, because "to be" and "to do" are different. Or are they? *Do what you will?*

"Whoever seeks Me must lose," He said. "To seek Me you must lose everything. To possess the fullness of life, you must submit and abandon all to My Heart, utterly. Stop asking Me why. I tell you now I will give you My joy to heal you a bit. And then you must submit to write about the one thing you have left, the apostolate to the handicapped. After that, you may know what I tell you," He said.

The daily Mass began. Five people were there. But, to me, the chapel was filled with so many other people. I looked at Him. He nodded.

"You're seeing it. You're believing it. Like that rite from St. John Chrysostom's Mass you have sung so often: 'We have seen the true faith. We have received the heavenly Spirit.' When you were converted by Me, you believed it all, and so you see: Don't be afraid. The Mass is when time and eternity meet."

To the left and to the right I saw the saints again, our friends, those whose names are known to all, those who have died that I know, and even those not yet born in time. God's children filled the room. I looked at the angels, so many in this one place. These large, invisible, rocklike beings are through and in and around this chapel. Surrounding the heads of the saints and some of the people there were various-colored auras that overwhelmed me. I felt like falling apart and did not. Those who see, see by faith.

At the consecration I watched Him in joy. My Lord! *O my God!* "I see that at this Mass, at every Mass, everywhere is You —You each time. A human priest, saying the words, and You take over in his voice whether he sees You or not. O Lord, please let them see You as You are, as the Spirit fills them. *Please?* Can't everyone see?"

Thank God, we could sing to release the tension in the memorial acclamation.

"Christ has died. Christ has risen. Christ will come again."

And I understood. What greater faith there is for those who do *not* see the Father, the Son, and the Holy Spirit, face to face.

"Through Him, with Him, in the Unity of the Holy Spirit all glory and honor are Yours, Almighty Father, for ever and ever. Amen."

In prayer, and in bliss of peace, I said with others, "Lord, I'm not worthy, but say Your Word and I shall be healed."

"I heal you daily," He said. "You are a mess and I love you. Now eat and drink and be silent, not knowing what to do. Be silent. Be still."

*Be still?* I'm not great at that when I have a job to do. And two opposites were crescendoing inside me in that coming week. As I understood it, my task was to delve into the meaning of my love in the apostolate of the handicapped, and to this end I was interviewing the members of the community.

And at the same time, "common sense" was snickering at me to explain the past six years of my life. "Common sense?" Do you know another name? I do not like using the show-off word "devil." I call him the Pretender. He's so suave, so insidious, that he makes us forget what is real. I tried to laugh him away.

I was making notes on the apostolate, which had opened on February 13, 1977. It encompasses not only those in wheelchairs but those of every age who accept the fact that they need to worship there. There, each is a helper and one in need of help. By newspaper, by parish bulletins, and by word of mouth, people learned in the diocese that this apostolate was dedicated to provide transportation within the university.

In my notes two things struck the core. Everyone there utterly loves being there. And everyone there is an "unusual person." That phrase of Viscardi captured the truth of this Mass. I knew that there was no earthly place I loved more than this weekly Mass at Sacred Heart. We, who need private prayer and meditation at home, also need a special community of worship and fellowship.

For this I was making notes and working. But, at the same time, I found myself looking at the dung heap of my life. The Pretender was interrupting in my mind. So finally I put aside my notes and faced him.

*Why in the world do you ever come back to Sacred Heart? You keep hitting your head against the wall. Go elsewhere. Do you know you are a failure? Get yourself some dignity and get out of here. You remind yourself and others that you are a failure. You're so proud of being a minister for the Eucharist. What for?*

"Because I love the place, and these people, and I'm privileged to be here," I said.

*Be practical. Six years ago you had your health, your marriage, your job, and your future. You fool! You praise God for that which was taken away?*

"Yes!"

*Look at yourself. You are now almost alone. You're divorced. You've got physical pain, mental anxiety, and spiritual problems. You worked hard for five years to get yourself back into life. And you lost it. You're a writer who can't spell. A teacher with no job. The future going down the toilet. Your so-called God has been trying to tell you something.*

My whole soul was sore. To touch my soul made me cringe. Security? Usefulness? Close human love? But my soul answered: "I'm not so bad off. There are people much worse off than I am. Don't be ridiculous."

Common sense laughed sarcastically. *You'll never make it. You're a nothing. How great is your God? For six years you've been playing a silly game. You and your prayer.*

*Suscipe!* One who sings prays twice, and then one can't hear the voice of the Pretender.

On Sunday, as I came to Mass, I was a little troubled. Looking over the past year of this apostolate, one pattern was clear. Each person insisted that the joy of our priest and their love for him was overwhelming. I, too, love him. But, as a journalist, I did not know how to handle that. If we were to help others start a similar handicapped group—Jewish, Protestant, or Catholic—it seemed proper to leave out the virtues of the shepherd. Yet, each person maintained that the love of this man exuberated from him, warming them in. The first time they came, they had been a little unsure. But, from then on, they felt it almost too good to be true.

"Angie said I ought to come here once. I didn't think it would be any good. But, the first day there, I felt wanted," said Steve Lazarecki. "I'd quit church. With my disease I wasn't forced to go to church in a wheelchair. When I came here I was so bitter, and feeling so sorry for myself! But suddenly I believed this Father loved me. That's what makes the difference."

Steve grabbed me closer to his wheelchair. "I want to be sure you understand what I'm saying. Look what Father did. As time went on, he sort of pushed me to read the epistle for Mass. He made me feel that I could. And when I made a mistake, nobody got mad. Here, every week, I feel that I'm having a real vacation with God, and I can face the rest of the week. My grown daughter saw a change in me. And she came here to bring a present of wine to Father for helping me. Do you know what he said to her? He said: 'I thank your father for letting me come to know *him*.' And then Father gave the wine to *me!*" Steve thought the priest was great. But I could see Steve was great too. Love helps love.

"You know, I feel humble in front of Father too," said Betty Marple. "The first time I came, it was he who brought me, and I was embarrassed, as a woman, because he had to carry me into the car. But a priest who would interrupt Mass to say, 'God bless you,' to a kid sneezing, shows me God is with us. And in his homily I lose myself in the presence of Jesus." I smiled. I felt humble before Betty's openness.

"Part of it is this priest. He is completely without malice or guile. When I first met him I was sure he had to be a phony. He isn't," said Anita Vigeant. I dared not giggle, but I suddenly realized that an honest compliment was a rebound. Anita has no guile, no phoniness to interfere, but a two-way acceptance of love in the priest.

Virginia Wieland butted in. "I'm handicapped, in a way. I've got a psychological hang-up on most churches. I see this community work. Listening to Father, who is with us, I always learn something. When my far-off friends come to visit, they wonder when I tell them we're going to the handicapped Mass. But after they go home they keep writing me, saying they wish they had such a priest. What else can I say?" And I was always learning something from Virginia, for she is building up the community and the priest.

"Now, wait a minute," said Pauline Matarazzo. "This one does have faults. He doesn't always talk loud enough!" She chuckled and I laughed, because we need to speak out on that.

"I do love him, but I think it isn't just he." I love her honesty, for she strengthens us all.

A serious student, John Majewski, nodded. "Father's a normal clergyman, thinking, doing, and saying what he ought to. Nothing strange, except that he isn't afraid to show love. He believes in us and trusts us, and we're so happy to respond. Together, here, people really get the message for him and for us. Here God can take over, and He does." And I surely respond to John and his insight.

That was the answer. Who is the Priest that thrills us? Who's the real Shepherd here? Not a human one whose homilies are too long, but the One from heaven and earth. And who makes this handicapped Mass so glorious? Why has He chosen us for this apostolate?

"You know," Patricia Kennedy sighed happily. "I think it's better because God feels comfortable with us!"

Her husband, Dan, wondered, "Is it because we're a small group? We hate large halls, but if this grew, if we had to meet in the café or the lounge, we'd still come and feel comfortable."

"I sure would," said Claire Testani.

Ken Boda was thinking. "Little Amy feels better here than in our regular parish."

"We're just lucky," said Maureen. "This Mass starts only when it's ready. We start around eleven. But Father waits till everybody's there. We're all relaxed because there is no hurry."

"That's it," Charlotte and Irv explained. "Parishes have to be punctual to make room for other Masses. We have a great privilege not to be hassled by time. After church it's almost two hours before people leave."

Carla Alter sat next to her guitar. "How simple life used to be in the early Church. But now, thank God, there are so many people in the Church over the world that time has to cause trouble. I'm just lucky to work at the handicapped Mass, not being regimented by the clock when I sing."

"Yup, a gift," said Steve Fitzpatrick.

"So God comforts me," said Ron Veilleux. "For that I'll stay handicapped forever."

Porter Cleveland, a handsome man with a cane, stood up. "Will you quit using the word handicapped as if it were the beginning and the end? I feel comfortable here, but it's time to go till next week. I'm worried about getting back to work, about money for my wife and children. You name it, I've got to look at the problems. And by ourselves, we're scared silly between the reprieve here. See ya!"

*Scared silly?* As we left, I suddenly looked at the inner faces of us all, a paradox of real joy confronting real terror. *My God,* I said, *we believe in joy. But we don't want to look at real terror.* Here, where there is respite, we are comforted by His people. But, as we leave, time grabs again with the mask of the Pretender. The community of the handicapped was a gift of love where time does not matter. But as I walked out with the others I looked at my own cane, and stopped. It looked like a staff. And I was carrying my bundles.

Passover?

Abruptly I went back alone to the chapel. At each Mass it is always Passover. Yet now I understood more. We were following the Lord's message. We had eaten and drunk. But as I sat, my staff I placed on the floor on one side, my bundles on the other, ready to go.

"Where are we going?" I whispered. I watched Him and I said, "I believe in You but I thought faith was more simple and serene. You are serene, but, by myself, I am not."

Suddenly, it was as if my bundle and my cane/staff were left up in the dunes. I was again a small child, holding His Hand, stepping into the sea, the water breaking gray-cold. There was a thunderstorm coming. As the breakers splashed over my face and I was falling, with nothing to hold on to with my toes, He held my hand. The deeper we went, the more I was confused, unknowing what creatures were under the sea. A horseshoe crab was swimming quickly past me. I was swallowing warm salt water, but as the breaker passed I could stand. And I laughed, looking up at Him. It felt awfully exciting! There was another, larger wave coming in, and He grabbed me and picked me up in His arms. Before the lightning, as the thunder rolled, He showed me a break through the late-afternoon light. In the fog mist there was a sunset, dark white brilliance. *Glory be to the Father!*

He turned, and we started back toward the beach, but instead He brought me deep blue-black rocks to sit on. *And to the Son. And to the Holy Spirit.* How warm His currents were!

He said: "Do you remember what you said to Me?" He asked, *"Suscipe?"*

"Take, O Lord, and receive my entire liberty, my memory, my understanding, and my whole will. All that I am and all I possess, You have given to me. I surrender it *all* to You—" I broke in. "What do you want with it?"

"Keep on."

"All to You, to dispose of according to Your Will. Give me only Your will and Your grace—" I stopped.

"Do you know what grace is?" He said. "It's not something outside you. Grace means 'mingling,' the mingling of divine and human. Humanly you are nothing. I am everything. All love is Mine. I mingle My love with all. I have tried so hard to tell each person how much I love them. To you, as much as you love Me, I am one with you. That's all that's necessary. Love Me, mingle with Me. That's what you were made for. That is what each child was made for, nothing more."

"But I'm still afraid, and I don't know why," I said.

"You love Me as deeply as you yet can. I'll hold you, and brace you, for you now need to know more.

"I taught you Babel first in aphasia, as a sign for all. To learn in time to be, someday, fused with eternity in My Word. Yes, a sign to be a child."

I looked at myself. He was always tranquil, and I was dripping, with sick gray and dark brown seaweed stuck on my clothes. And He picked it off and cleaned me, and I was dry.

"I taught you that Babel of the human condition. Yes, a sign. But be braced close to Me, and do not be afraid."

I sat there beside Him in the darkness. The moon, everything, was gone.

"In eternity I am, in the beginning, now, and forever, the Son of God, Three-in-One. But in time I have been lonely all My life, confounded by Babel. Time is the Cross, from birth to death—and beyond. In time did I know who I was? Yes, and no. No human beings know for sure on earth. But you know time is often horrible.

"From the time that I was conceived I knew in eternity that I accepted sin. So everywhere I knew contradictions against contradictions.

"See Babel with Joseph and My Mother and Me? My Father wanted Me in the Temple, and I obeyed. Obedience—to whom? *Honor your father and mother!* Mine were worried when I seemed to disobey them, and they were afraid of not finding Me. I had lived under their obedience as a son. Yet they were living in obedience too. And from the Temple I went home again under their authority. People make simple things complex. The Father's will is Mine, and We are so simple. Only love can translate it. 'Love God, and do what you will.'"

That's what it means, being human, I thought. And I knew that my own faith alone is useless. I pulled myself closer to Him. I really wanted to go to sleep.

"But, child, you have to face terror! I teach you now the Babel of terror, the sign of your age!" He stood, saying where I could hardly see Him, "Anxiety breathes from the Leviathan, his flame singeing My people." He crouched down with me. "Read My gospel. From My Joseph to Saul, and always from Me, a prayer to the Father in the confounding of Babel in our heads.

"But brace yourself. Stand up! So often you have thought of Me on the Cross. But, child! That was *not* the end. Listen and remember! I died—and I descended into hell. Chaos! *Chaos!*"

His voice was the most horrible cry I ever dreamed of, nightmare beyond nightmare. The fear in me was unbearable. But I saw Him and I would not hide or run away. Oh, God, I saw hell, for I would go with Him. His cry? As a child newly born cries, I heard the anguish no words can explain. I heard His cry as He died on Golgotha. But then went further as He braced me at His side.

"Suffering Servant, I must go through the abyss of chaos, the total, total hell. Where is the house of light? See, I fall and fall to the cornerstone. I give all!" No sign. *No sound. Nothing!*

"There! I am slaughtered, holocausted by Myself, to share My flesh and My blood, the new passover Lamb. I die, split in half. And then, only then, do I see Him."

I had fallen within Him, falling as if even faith and hope were suspended, while love sounded more like blasphemy over the abyss. To hear the word, the Body and the Blood of the Living God? Terrible? Ah, yes. The terrible loving God, so simple that till then I had not accepted it. So seldom do we know the word "terrible," so sweet.

Thank God, I could not see but only hear the voices of the Pretender, common sense. Hell is full of his teaching that the real God could not be His way.

He, the Lamb, and the Shepherd at once, showed us the Three-in-One. Just past hell is eternity, next door.

I opened my eyes and I knew I had been there before. Again the soundless song, the majesty and the sweetness, the body, mind, and soul exulting in raptures.

He raised me back to the rock. Off the dunes I could see my cane and my bundle. My mouth was open, speechless.

"You have seen Me. And you have seen hell. You were not ready to accept all of life. Your illness was not merely your disability or aphasia or being handicapped. Your disease was that you had to learn and integrate Us who made you all. Where have you been? With My Love you have rejoiced in goodness, but *good* is too overwhelming to encounter love. You have seen the terror. Anxiety has been part of your life, accepting but not seeing that that, too, is the One.

"I am the Resurrection and the Life. But there is no proof. Just Me. And each person must will to believe. I who came. I who love. I who die. I who rise. I who return . . . *Do you believe?*"

"Oh, God, yes! I do believe," I said.

"Tell those who are afraid, I am with them. For those who do not believe in Me, they see Me as a failure. But I am the judge. Many who do not see Me may believe Me more than those who pretend to love Me.

"You are a fool to love Me. But I am the greatest fool of all, for I love so much that I continually come to save you all. Peace? Peace is not as you thought it to be. Peace is not placid. Peace is integrating opposites, spiraling, moving, creating.

"In peace will you take the kiss of Judas as well as the kiss of the Song of Songs? For both are Mine."

I said, "I hope I will not ask any more: 'What will tomorrow bring?' I'll just be. Keep me a fool to be continued, I pray, to the end."